A LITTLE BOOK OF SELF CARE

BREATHWORK

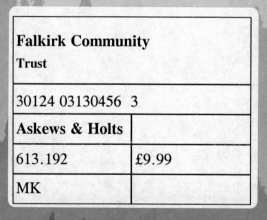

A LITTLE BOOK OF SELF CARE

BREATHWORK

USE THE POWER OF BREATH TO ENERGIZE
YOUR BODY AND FOCUS YOUR MIND

NATHALIA WESTMACOTT-BROWN

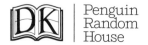

Senior Editors Lesley Malkin, Rona Skene
Senior Designer Collette Sadler
Designer Philippa Nash
Editorial Assistant Kiron Gill
Illustrator Mikyung Lee
Producer, Pre-production Heather Blagden
Senior Producer Luca Bazzoli
Jacket Designer Amy Cox
Jacket Co-ordinator Lucy Philpott
Creative Technical Support
Sonia Charbonnier
Managing Editor Dawn Henderson
Managing Art Editor Marianne Markham
Art Director Maxine Pedliham
Publishing Director Mary-Clare Jerram

First published in Great Britain in 2019 by
Dorling Kindersley Limited
80 Strand, London WC2R 0RL

DISCLAIMER see page 144

A CIP catalogue record for this book is available
from the British Library.
ISBN: 978-0-2413-8455-8

Printed and bound in China

A WORLD OF IDEAS:
SEE ALL THERE IS TO KNOW

www.dk.com

CONTENTS

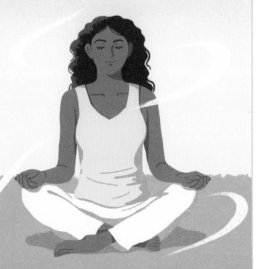

FOREWORD

We live in a world where health advice is cheap. On TV, on social media or in magazines, all kinds of doctors, celebrities and self-styled experts are telling us what we need to do: stop drinking, smoking, medicating, stressing, over-working, or eating the wrong things. But for many of us, business goes on as usual, until something drastic happens.

My life-changing event was a high-speed motorway crash, following a period of overwork and burnout in the film production industry. I am eternally grateful that nobody was injured or killed, but as I lay face-down on the grass, surrounded by wreckage, I clearly remember thinking, "This is it. Something has to change."

That experience in 1999 prompted me to quit my job and begin a spiritual quest that has lasted nearly two decades, taking me all over the world to learn about a then little-known practice called breathwork. I am blessed to have been apprenticed to some inspirational breathwork teachers, and after all that, I am even more convinced of what I suspected in the first place... the ultimate health solution I was searching for was right under my nose all along! Breathing consciously, also known as breathwork, offers a chance to experience unbelievable physical, psychological and spiritual transformation. This book is your way to tap into this effective and fast-growing area of natural healthcare.

Scientific research is now proving what yogis and mystics have known for thousands of years. This simple, invisible force – the breath – can improve brain function, decision-making, physical capabilities, endurance levels, and even induce profound transpersonal meditative states.

This book of self care is an opportunity for you to start to explore the exciting world of breathwork. To make it really easy, the exercises are divided into Physical, Psychological, Spiritual, and First-aid interventions so you can easily find the page you need. You don't need special equipment or a specific location; many exercises can be safely practised anywhere – at home, in the office, or while you wait for your order at the coffee shop.

The exercises are organized to correspond with specific symptoms, but don't wait for a health crisis to benefit from conscious breathing. Breathwork will help you to maintain as well as regain your health. Try all the exercises, then practise the ones that work for you.

My sincere hope is that you will carry this book around to help you develop a happy, healthy relationship with your breath. Optimum breathing is optimum living. For those who wish to journey deeper, there is an increasing number of teachers and practitioners who are trained to guide you into a new relationship with breath and life. You'll find information on how to find those people in the resources section, at the back of the book.

Enjoy the ride – may you breathe as if your life depends upon it!

With love always,

Nathalia Westmacott-Brown

BREATHWORK

BEGINNINGS

THE POWER OF BREATH

It's safe to say that if you are reading this book, you have already mastered the art of breathing for survival! What many of us do not realize however, is that the breath, when trained through breathwork, can also connect us to profound personal and transpersonal experiences. For some, this will be a powerful voyage into the emotions; for others, it is experienced as a spiritual journey. But what all breathworkers agree upon is that becoming breath-conscious is an inspirational gateway to feeling truly alive. Breathe fully and deeply with awareness to empower the body, focus the mind, and nourish the spirit.

Significant reduction in anxiety; improved motivation; greater focus; improved creativity; better communication.

More positive body image; improved immune functioning; better circulation; decrease in physical pain.

Greater physical strength and stamina; reduction in muscle tension; greater freedom of movement.

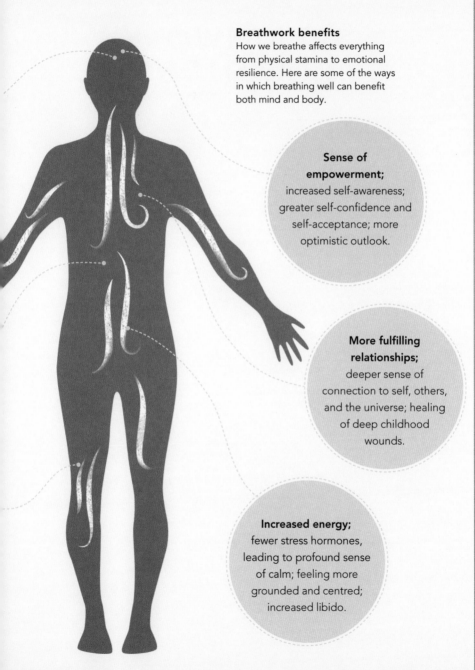

Breathwork benefits

How we breathe affects everything
from physical stamina to emotional
resilience. Here are some of the ways
in which breathing well can benefit
both mind and body.

**Sense of
empowerment;**
increased self-awareness;
greater self-confidence and
self-acceptance; more
optimistic outlook.

**More fulfilling
relationships;**
deeper sense of
connection to self, others,
and the universe; healing
of deep childhood
wounds.

Increased energy;
fewer stress hormones,
leading to profound sense
of calm; feeling more
grounded and centred;
increased libido.

BREATHWORK TRADITIONS

Breathwork encompasses a wealth of traditions, modalities, and practices both ancient and modern, and from all parts of the world. Here is a flavour of the major influences on the breathwork exercises in this book. If you want to find out more, there is a list of references to major breathwork modalities and schools on pages 138–139.

PRANAYAMA/KRIYA YOGA/TANTRA
RELIGION Hinduism
ORIGIN India

Pranayama is an ancient yogic discipline involving breath and body postures, and is the fourth of the eight branches of Ashtanga Yoga. "Prana" means life force, and "ayama" indicates "to extend or draw out" as in extension of the life force.

DAO YIN/QIGONG
RELIGION Buddhism
ORIGIN South-east Asia

This breath and movement practice gently balances your "qi" energy (also known as "chi"), revitalizes body, mind, and spirit, and develops physical strength and flexibility.

COHERENT BREATH
FOUNDER Stephen Elliott
ORIGIN USA

This method uses a measured breathing rate of 5 breaths per minute. The process maximizes heart rate variability (HRV), which has a positive effect on circulation and improves the overall health of the body.

BUTEYKO BREATHING
FOUNDER: Dr. Konstantin Buteyko
ORIGIN: Russia

This method is based on the concept that "over-breathing" is the underlying cause of many medical conditions. Buteyko promotes nasal breathing, reduced breathing and relaxation.

INTEGRATIVE BREATHWORK
FOUNDER Jacquelyn Small
ORIGIN USA

This process combines conscious breathing with other powerful healing methods. Integrative breathwork responds to the needs of the client, with a range of interventions that have conscious breath at their core. Practitioners may use breath with art processes, Gestalt psychology, neuro-linguistic programming (NLP), visualisation, bodywork, and nature rituals.

REBIRTHING BREATHWORK
FOUNDER Leonard Orr
ORIGIN USA

Rebirthing evolved in the 1970s in California as a result of altered states of consciousness exploration. Leonard Orr experimented with breathing in hot water and found that breath can surface deep memories as far back as the womb and birth experience. He asserted that clearing the trauma around the first breath was central to a healthy breathing pattern.

MIDDENDORF BREATHWORK
FOUNDER Professor Ilse Middendorf
ORIGIN Germany

In 1935 Professor Ilse Middendorf evolved a form of breath education based on connecting with the natural breath. Her approach offers "a conscious experience of the sensation of movement of breath, free from control of the human will".

HOLOGRAPHIC BREATHWORK
FOUNDER Martin Jones
ORIGIN United Kingdom

Whilst battling a life-threatening illness in 2002, Martin Jones discovered a profound meditative breath practice which he called Holographic Breathing. This method not only healed his Lyme Disease, but has proven effective for a range of conditions including insomnia, asthma, pain, and chronic fatigue.

BREATHWORK PREPARATION

This book offers a range of breathing exercises and processes that can be safely undertaken at home, and are designed to support you as you face physical, psychological, emotional, or spiritual challenges. Here's how to prepare your mind and body to get the most out of your practice.

HEALTH CONCERNS

Some of the dynamic exercises in this book are not advisable for everyone. If you are living with a health condition, are pregnant, or have any concerns about your state of health, please exercise self-responsibility by:

• Asking your doctor/health professional if breathing exercises are appropriate for you.

• Listening and working within the limitations of your body in the moment.

• Starting slowly and working up to longer sessions.

• Finding a qualified breath worker to provide you with the additional support you need.

If you are in any doubt, check with a health professional before you start!

STATE YOUR INTENTIONS

In breathwork, we aim to move beyond mere survival breath to a breathing pattern that is accompanied by awareness. Breathing consciously means observing (and sometimes changing) our breath pattern with a particular intention – for example, "I am going to breathe for more energy", or "this session is all about letting go".

THINK ABOUT POSTURE

Your breath exercises will be most effective when your body is comfortable and your respiratory system is open, with your spine straight but relaxed. If a suggested position isn't right for you, adjust it until you feel comfortable. A relaxed body breathes more fully and realigns more easily than a tense one.

CHOOSE NOSE OR MOUTH

There is a breath for all occasions. Experiment with both nose and mouth breathing to open up the fullest range of experiences and feelings in the body. Generally, breathing through the nose is calming and balancing, whereas mouth breathing is energizing and promotes emotional release.

EFFECTIVE POSTURES

- **Sitting in a chair** – keep your spine straight and your feet flat on the ground.

- **Kneeling or cross-legged** – ensure your body is relaxed, with no pressure on the legs.

- **Standing** – take care standing for dynamic exercises as you can feel dizzy at first.

- **Walking** – it can be helpful to synchronize the rhythm of your steps and breaths.

OTHER PHYSICAL POSITIONS

- **Prayer position** – many exercises end with the hands in the "prayer" position over the heart. This is not a religious gesture, but a simple act of completion and balancing of left and right.

- **Chin tucked down** – this is a slight downwards tilt which opens the back of the neck, enabling better connection between brain and body.

BREATHWORK PRACTICE

Breathwork exercises can benefit you in virtually any situation, but for the best effects, make a commitment to practise them regularly over a period of time. Each exercise in this book has specific instructions, but here are some general principles to follow, to ensure you get the most from your practice. Above all, listen to your body and always take your time.

01

START BY OBSERVING

Begin by simply watching your breathing, without making any changes, for a few inhales and exhales. This raises your consciousness of where you are in the moment. Breath combined with consciousness leads to transformation… and consciousness means noticing what's going on right now.

02

LISTEN TO YOUR BODY

Just as thoughts are the mind's voice, feelings are the body's means of expression. Whatever you feel during an exercise, try to accept the sensation, even if you are not enjoying it much. Your feelings are not inherently dangerous. It is safe to feel!

03

FIND A RHYTHM

There are recommendations on rhythm and pace in the exercises, but always listen to the needs of your body and go more slowly if you need to. The more natural the process feels, the more likely you are to enter into an altered, enhanced state of awareness.

04

COUNT YOUR BREATHS

Counting the length of the inhales or exhales or the number of breaths in a cycle can help you evolve a natural rhythm, but always listen to your body and adjust recommended counts if you need to. Breathing practice is not competitive. Consistent awareness is far more important than Olympic-level breathing cycles.

05

STAY GROUNDED

Breathing consciously can unleash intense emotion and high energy levels that can feel overwhelming. If this happens, come out of the process gradually – slow the breathing and shift to nose breath for a calming effect. Take up a grounded position, such as lying on your side. Consider breathing with a practitioner for additional support and sense of safety.

06

COMPLETE THE PROCESS

Breathwork is a form of self-healing, so it is fitting to begin and end your process with conscious intention. Open your exercises with silent observation and close with a physical gesture of completion, such as bringing the hands together over the heart.

CONSCIOUS CONNECTED BREATHING

Conscious connected breathing (CCB) forms part of many of the exercises in this book. It brings a constant flow of energy into the body for the purpose of healing, and counteracts the muscular shrinkage associated with sub-ventilation (not using enough of your lung capacity), by encouraging an open breathing movement. The pace is slightly faster than normal, but without forcing or pushing. Your breathing, which you will hear faintly, keeps awareness focused on your body experience rather than in the mind/thought process.

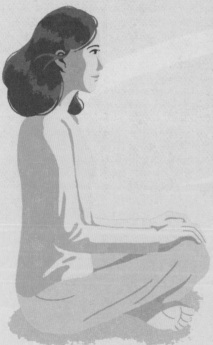

BREATH OF LIFE

Ancient breathwork traditions such as Dao Yin and pranayama teach that when we breathe consciously we are not only taking in oxygen but also breathing "prana", "life force", or "qi" energy into the body. This is the essential energy that activates healing and wellness.

Healing energy

Bringing awareness to our breath – noticing and potentially changing the pattern that we are in – can bring great benefits to body and mind.

THE PROCESS

Conscious connected breathing involves eliminating the pause between the inhale and the exhale, and breathing in and out through your nose or your mouth in a continuous motion of breath.

01

Find an open and relaxed position for your body. Slightly tuck your chin towards your chest.

02

Choose to breathe either through your mouth or your nose. Begin to breathe with no pause between the inhale and the exhale.

03

Make the inhale longer – breathe in for 2–3 seconds and out for about a second. Focus on the in-breath, releasing the exhale naturally, without effort. To encourage this soft exhale, you can add a little sigh as you breathe out.

04

Breathe in this pattern for a few minutes, moving your body as little as possible and noticing any different sensations arising.

05

Place a hand on your abdomen. Allow your breath to move your hand. Then raise your hand to the diaphragm and mid-rib area. Feel your breath moving your hand here. Lift your hand to the chest area. Notice how your hand rises and falls with your breath.

06

After a few minutes, shift the pattern so that inhales and exhales are now of equal length, or if you prefer, you can make the exhale longer. Notice that this shift of emphasis has the effect of calming down any stimulating feelings.

07

Practise this technique when you need to build either stimulation and action, or calm energy and peaceful integration in the body. The process also opens up breathing areas that have become closed or inactive.

BREATH
PRACTICES

PHYSICAL SELF

Simple breath control can have an immediate, significant, and lasting effect on so many aspects of physical wellbeing – from reducing painful symptoms, to helping the body's systems work better, improving sleep, and boosting your energy levels.

OBSERVING YOUR BREATHING

To address physical, emotional, or spiritual growth through breathwork, it is important to create a regular space to notice what your breath is doing. Zen meditation uses breath counting, a process that involves counting slow inhalations and exhalations, and this can help you to be present in the moment.

02

Begin breath counting by counting "1" to yourself as you breathe out. Lengthen the next out-breath, counting "1, 2," then breathe in again.

01

Take a few deep breaths in and out through the nose, then let your breath return to its natural pattern. Under normal circumstances, this should be gentle and slow.

NEED TO KNOW

BENEFITS Focus, clarity, concentration, and relaxation; provides the foundation for breath exercises.

TIME 5–10 minutes; daily.

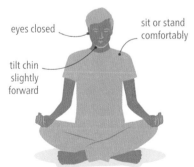

eyes closed

sit or stand comfortably

tilt chin slightly forward

03

As you next exhale, count "1, 2, 3," and so on until you reach a count of 5 on the out-breath.

04

On the next out-breath, exhale for a count of 1, then repeat steps 2–3, building up to a count of 5 and then starting the cycle again at 1.

05

If your attention wanders, simply start again, counting "1" on the next out-breath. Continue for at least 5 minutes. Open your eyes and return to your day.

GAUGING BREATH CAPACITY

Unless you are an opera singer or athlete, you probably don't know your breath capacity. Many of us have poor breathing patterns and underuse our capacity to take in life-giving air. This "Control Pause" test, evolved by Dr Buteyko, will give you an insight into your breathing. Then turn to pages 28–29 for ways to increase your breath capacity.

NEED TO KNOW

BENEFITS Increases awareness; informs next steps for your breath practice.

TIME 1–2 minutes.

EQUIPMENT Clock or stop-watch.

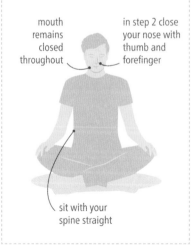

mouth remains closed throughout

in step 2 close your nose with thumb and forefinger

sit with your spine straight

01

Sit comfortably with your spine straight. Breathe in a natural rhythm through your nose for 30 seconds.

02

Take a regular breath in and out. Then gently close your nose and count the seconds until you feel the need to breathe in. Allow the nose to gently open again and take a breath through the nose.

03

The number of seconds you count is your Control Pause. The longer the pause, the better your overall health is likely to be. Check your Control Pause before and after exercise to see if there is an increase in capacity.

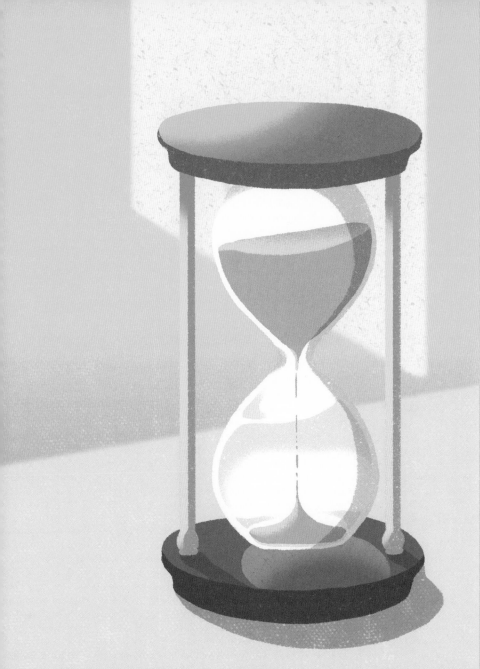

INCREASING BREATH CAPACITY

This is a great daily stress-busting exercise you can do anywhere without anyone knowing. It relieves shallow breathing caused by stress and poor posture. Known as the Three-part Breath, this soothing pranayama exercise opens up the breathing centres in the belly, diaphragm/ribcage, and chest.

NEED TO KNOW

BENEFITS Helps shortness of breath, sub-ventilation, anxiety, and palpitations; reduces stress and improves focus.

TIME 5–10 minutes daily/as needed.

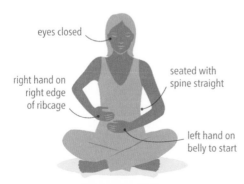

eyes closed

right hand on right edge of ribcage

seated with spine straight

left hand on belly to start

02

As you breathe in, feel your belly lift naturally, followed by the expansion of your ribs. As you breathe out, feel the slight contraction of your ribs, followed by the drop of your belly. Breathe out fully.

01

Close your eyes and relax your face and body, while breathing naturally through your nose. Bring your awareness to your breath as it moves gently in and out of your body.

03

Now position your
right hand in the centre of your
chest, just below your collarbone.
Lengthen your in-breath so it
opens the belly, then the ribs,
then arrives in the chest. Notice
your hands lifting and falling
with the wave of breath.

04

Continue observing this
wave at your own pace: inhale
in 3 parts (belly lifts, ribs expand,
and chest rises); and exhale in
3 parts (chest drops, ribs contract,
and belly softens and falls).
Do not pause between the
inhale and exhale.

05

Relax your arms
and focus entirely on your
breath, keeping the 3-part
wave moving up and down the
body. After 20 connected
breaths, return to normal
breathing.

02

When you are ready, close your eyes and soften your jaw, taking your awareness inward. Focus on nose breathing and slow it down: deep, rhythmic breaths will gradually relax your body.

01

Lying on your back, become aware of all parts of your body and invite relaxation with light stretching. If you need to, adjust your position so that you are completely comfortable.

RETURNING TO SELF

This hatha yoga practice is useful for bringing you into balance when you feel scattered. It reconnects you to your body and your breath, teaching you to listen to the subtle cues and signals from the body that help you to relax. Although you are lying down, this is a fully conscious pose, in which you can practise being awake, yet totally relaxed.

03

As you inhale through your nose, be aware of the breath as it fills your lungs. Notice that your abdomen rises. Without pause, exhale through your nose; your abdomen will fall naturally as air leaves your lungs.

04

Let rhythmic breathing take over as the inhale and exhale flow into one another. Continue for as long as you can maintain awareness of how you react to the process. When you are ready to finish, roll over and come into an upright position.

NEED TO KNOW

BENEFITS Rejuvenation; improved circulation; better posture; sense of calm.

TIME 5–10 minutes or as long as needed; daily or as needed.

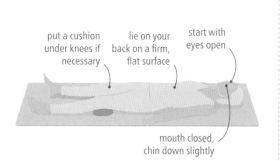

put a cushion under knees if necessary

lie on your back on a firm, flat surface

start with eyes open

mouth closed, chin down slightly

RELEASING TENSION

Try tantric breathing to relieve physical or mental tension and bring you to a sense of connection with yourself, in turn leaving you open and ready to connect with others. Conscious breathing is a central part of this deep, sensual exercise, which is practised to awaken, invigorate, and release your own life-force energy for the purpose of self-healing.

02

Drop your jaw a little and inhale deeply through your mouth, while expanding your belly outwards.

NEED TO KNOW

BENEFITS Relaxation; softness in the body; receptivity; trust, clarity, and connection.

TIME 5 minutes or as long as needed; daily.

01

Invite relaxation into your body and observe your breathing (see pages 24–25) for 3–5 breaths.

sit or lie down comfortably

eyes closed

mouth open a little

03

Breathe out deeply through
your mouth, allowing your
belly to drop back inwards.
Accompany the exhale
with a long gentle "Aah"
sound for a count of 5.

04

Continue this gentle,
open-mouthed belly-breathing,
sighing on the exhale. Now
invite each sigh to gently
release whatever is causing
tension within your body
and/or mind.

05

When you are ready,
let the last of your tension
go on a final out-breath,
leaving you more receptive to
those around you. End with
a gesture of completion
(see page 15).

COMBATING FATIGUE

This conscious, connected mouth-breathing process combats fatigue and inertia and brings the breather back to joy, inspiration, and energy. A Transformational Breath® process, it is ideal when you know what you need to do to stay healthy, but can't raise the energy to do it. Afterwards, with renewed willpower, improve your wellbeing with a run or a healthy meal.

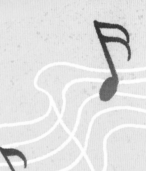

01

Start the music, and bring your awareness to your breathing. Relax your jaw and open your mouth wide so you can breathe in and out through your mouth without straining.

NEED TO KNOW

BENEFITS Energized body-mind; clarity, drive, focus, willpower, and motivation.

TIME 3–5 minutes.

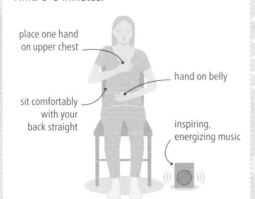

place one hand on upper chest

hand on belly

sit comfortably with your back straight

inspiring, energizing music

02

Start counting each complete breath. Breathe smoothly, with no gap between the inhale and exhale, until you have counted 100 breaths. Feel uplifted by both breath and music.

03

Now say out loud some positive affirmations while breathing consciously (see pages 18–19): "I am worthy to receive energy"; "I embrace this day"; "It is natural for me to move forward with grace and ease."

04

Now take a deep breath in and hold it for 3–5 seconds, then gently release it. Complete the process by bringing your hands to the prayer position in front of your heart.

05

Close your eyes for a moment. If you feel light-headed, remain seated until you feel grounded. Then stand up slowly.

CALMING YOUR NERVES

Ocean breath is an effective way to rebalance your body, mind, and spirit when you are feeling nervous. In this gentle breathing cycle, you use a slight contraction in the throat to recreate the soothing, whooshing sound of waves which, with practice, will calm both body and mind. Helpful any time, ocean breath is particularly beneficial when you cannot sleep.

02

When you are comfortable making this sound on the exhale, hold the slight contraction while inhaling too, making a wave-like sound as your breath moves gently in and out.

01

Breathe in through your mouth and as you breathe out, slightly contract the back of your throat, softly whispering "Huhh". Avoid contracting too much, which will tighten the throat.

NEED TO KNOW

BENEFITS Calm mind; warm, energized body; and present-moment awareness.

TIME 5 minutes daily; building up over time.

CAUTION Seek guidance if you have a respiratory condition such as COPD or asthma. Slow down if you feel faint or dizzy.

eyes closed

slightly open mouth, relaxed jaw and tongue

hands on your knees, palms up

03

Close your mouth,
keeping your lips soft and
your tongue relaxed. As you
breathe through your nose,
keep up both the contraction
and the wave sound from the
back of your throat.

04

Now, focus completely
on the sound of your breath,
which should be audible
only to you, letting it calm
you. Breathe rhythmically
and smoothly.

05

Fill your lungs as much as
possible without straining, then
fully release the breath as you
breathe out. Continue for as
long as it feels comfortable
before returning to a normal
breathing pattern.

BOOSTING YOUR RESILIENCE

Wim Hof earned the nickname "Ice Man" through spectacular feats of physical endurance. He devised the Wim Hof Method® to build the ability to withstand cold, heat, and fear. Conscious breathing is a key tool of the method, popular with those looking to harness and hone their inner power to endure physical and psychological challenges.

02

Now inhale deeply, completely filling your lungs. Release that breath through your mouth and hold without breathing in for as long as you can, without straining.

NEED TO KNOW

BENEFITS Cardiovascular health and good circulation; wellbeing; access to inner power.

TIME 5–10 minutes.

CAUTION Avoid if you have any history of epilepsy; high blood pressure; heart disease; stroke.

mouth open

chin slightly turned down

sit comfortably with back straight

leave at least two hours after a meal

01

Breathe in and out through your mouth in short, strong breaths, as if blowing up a balloon. Repeat 30 times, keeping a steady rhythmic pace and using your abdomen fully.

03

When you feel the need, gently breathe in fully through your mouth. Hold your breath at the top of the inhale for around 10 seconds, then release it. Repeat this process twice, so that you complete 3 breath cycles in total.

04

Relax your body and notice how it feels. You may feel light-headed and tingly – this is due to taking in more oxygen than usual. With practice, the exercise can leave you feeling meditative.

05

If you feel light-headed, remain seated until you feel more grounded. Take your time before standing up slowly and returning to your day.

COLD-WATER SYSTEM BOOST

People have long used conscious breathwork with cold-water immersion as an invigorating health maintenance process. Daily cold-water showering is simple, powerful, and effective – or, for a weekly system boost, find a safe local lake or river in which to immerse yourself. If that isn't feasible, make a home ice bath – simply add a few bags of ice to a bath of cold water.

01

At the end of your normal shower, turn down the temperature as low as you can manage. Begin to breathe consciously (see pages 18–19) through your mouth.

02

Stay under the cold water for as long as you can, continuing to mouth-breathe. Don't worry if you can only manage a minute or less at first.

NEED TO KNOW

BENEFITS Improves circulation; reduces muscle inflammation; induces a sense of wellbeing and stamina; reduces cellulite.

TIME Start with 1–3 minutes, and work up.

CAUTION Not suitable for those with epilepsy, high blood pressure, heart disease, or when pregnant.

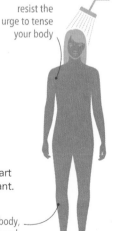

resist the urge to tense your body

your whole body, including your head, should be wet

03

Try to allow the water to run over your whole head and body so there is no resistance, tension or holding back. You should find that your initial resistance shifts after about 20 seconds as your skin adjusts to the cold.

04

Gradually increase your time until you can stay in the cold water for 3–5 minutes. Focus completely on your breathing, by taking big, deep, controlled breaths.

02

As you breathe out, flatten your lower belly. The area just below your belly button gets pulled up, in, and back a little way towards your lower back ribs.

01

Breathe normally through your nose. Direct your next in-breath towards your tailbone, inhaling up the back of your ribs, lifting your lower ribs away from your hips.

REDUCING BACK PAIN

With practice, this back-breathing exercise from the Pilates tradition can improve your posture and reduce or even eliminate back pain. This process cultivates space between the bones of the back and elongates the curve of the spine. It offers support to lower abdominal muscles and reduces neck and shoulder tension.

03

As you continue to exhale, roll your shoulders back and down to lengthen your upper back and extend your head and neck lightly upwards. This completes one breathing cycle.

04

Repeat steps 1–3 for at least 5 minutes; longer will be beneficial. It might feel odd at first but with practice, you will find a rhythm. Return to normal breathing. If you were lying or sitting down, get up slowly.

NEED TO KNOW

BENEFITS Pain reduction; improved posture; elongated spine; easier breathing.

TIME 5–10 minutes, regularly through the day; as needed.

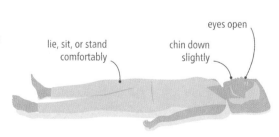

lie, sit, or stand comfortably

chin down slightly

eyes open

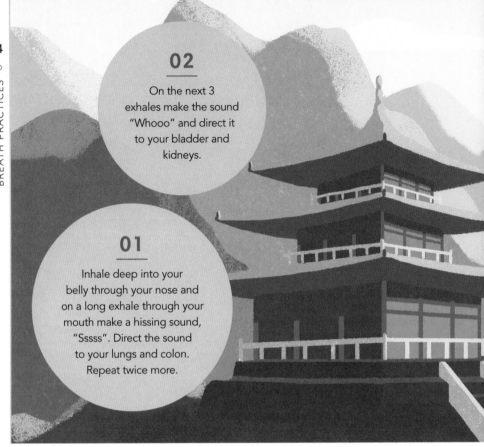

02

On the next 3 exhales make the sound "Whooo" and direct it to your bladder and kidneys.

01

Inhale deep into your belly through your nose and on a long exhale through your mouth make a hissing sound, "Sssss". Direct the sound to your lungs and colon. Repeat twice more.

STRENGTHEN YOUR CORE

If you're feeling stressed and out of balance, this simple Taoist exercise will soothe your emotions and support your core by focusing on your inner organs, where negative energy is stored. The six healing exhalations, each repeated at least three times, use sound-toning together with your breath to harmonize your body and mind.

03

Now exhale the sound "Shhh" 3 times, directing it to your liver and gall bladder. On the next 3 exhales make a "Haaaa" sound, directing it to your heart and small intestine.

04

Then exhale a gutteral "Wooo" in the back of your throat and direct it to your spleen and stomach. Repeat twice more.

05

Finally, hiss the sound "Heee" through your teeth, 3 times, to harmonize the energy and flow of your body. Finish by bringing your hands together and thanking the energies you worked with.

NEED TO KNOW

BENEFITS Harmonized emotional and physical health.

TIME 2–3 minutes daily or as often as needed.

any comfortable position, standing or seated

mouth closed to start, then open to make sound

spine straight

ACCESSING SEXUAL ENERGY

Gain clarity about how open or closed you feel sexually through open-mouth tantric breathing, either alone or with a trusted partner. Tantric traditions help you to connect with your sexual or life-force energy, using breath, movement, and sound to explore your experience in a shame-free, tender, and loving way. Stay comfortable, proceeding slowly with consideration.

01

Drop your jaw open and inhale deeply through your mouth, expanding your belly, then exhale deeply, letting your belly drop back. Take 3–5 open-mouth breaths in this way.

NEED TO KNOW

BENEFITS Increased connection with self and others; release of repressed emotions.

TIME 5 minutes daily; building up over time.

CAUTION This dynamic process may not be suitable for pregnant women or those with lower back pain.

lie on a firm surface such as a yoga mat

close your eyes or gaze softly at the ceiling

Lie on your back with palms facing up

tilt your chin slightly down to your chest

02

Once breathing like this feels natural, add sound by accompanying each exhale with a long gentle "Aah". Repeat, making the sound on the exhale until it feels rhythmic and natural.

03

Keep the belly breath and sounds going. Bend your knees so your feet are flat on the ground, hip-width apart. Roll your arms to palms-down on the floor.

04

On your next inhale, push through your hands and feet to lift your pelvis up a few inches. Exhale with the "Aah" sound and lower your pelvis back to the ground. Repeat, inhaling as you lift the pelvis and exhaling as you lower it.

05

When breath, sound, and movement are all synchronized, continue for a few minutes. Then breathe normally and roll on to your side to finish.

PSYCHOLOGICAL SELF

Many doctors and psychotherapists now recognize that, in addition to the clear physical benefits, optimal breathing plays a vital role in helping to keep our psychological and emotional capabilities fluid and responsive.

OVERCOMING A BUSY MIND

When time is short and your mind is scattered, Alternate Nostril Breathing, an ancient pranayama exercise that balances the right and left hemispheres of your brain, calms anxiety and clears your head. This is useful when you are studying or before an important meeting, when you need focused mental capabilities.

02

At the top of the in-breath, close your left nostril with your ring finger and lift your thumb to release your right nostril. Breathe out slowly through your right nostril for a count of 4.

NEED TO KNOW

BENEFITS Mental clarity; increased discipline; increased attention span.

TIME 5–10 minutes, or as long as you feel relaxed and comfortable.

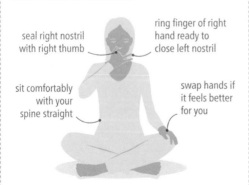

ring finger of right hand ready to close left nostril

seal right nostril with right thumb

sit comfortably with your spine straight

swap hands if it feels better for you

01

When you are ready, close your right nostril with your right thumb. Inhale through your left nostril for a count of 4.

03

Keeping the left nostril closed, breathe in through your right nostril to the count of 4. Close the right nostril with your thumb, release the left nostril, and breathe out. This completes a set.

04

Continue with another set, this time breathing in and out to the count of 5. Keep your breath steady, rhythmic, and smooth, without straining. Lengthen each set by one count, building up to a count of 8.

05

Repeat the process 5–10 times, completing at the end of a set. To finish, close your eyes and bring your hands to prayer.

01

Breathe consciously through
your nose (see pages
18–19). Rest your tongue on
the roof of your mouth and
tuck the tip behind your
teeth. Bend your knees
a little.

03

Keep this motion going for a
few more breaths: on the
in-breath, let your wrists gently
guide your arms upwards; on
the out-breath, let your wrists
take your arms back down to
your belly area.

02

On the inhale, gently lift your
arms upwards in front of your
body, leading with your wrists. At
the top of the in-breath, when
your wrists are shoulder height,
softly and slowly change direction,
sweeping your arms gently down
as you exhale.

SEPARATING FROM DISTRACTIONS

If you find yourself lacking focus, use this simple breath and body
exercise to anchor your awareness in the present moment and release
your mind from unwanted distractions. With regular practice, this
slow and relaxed exercise, based on the ancient Chinese practice of
Dao Yin, will offer you access to a deep meditative state.

05

Continue this practice for a few minutes and when you feel ready, bring your hands softly into the prayer position as a gesture of closure and balance.

04

On the in-breath, gently straighten your knees as your arms go up. On the out-breath, gently bend your knees as your arms come down. Bring total mindfulness to these movements: synchronize your knees, arms, and breath, so they all rise on the inhale and fall on the exhale.

NEED TO KNOW

BENEFITS Centred in self; body and mind integrated and in harmony.

TIME 5 minutes or as long as possible.

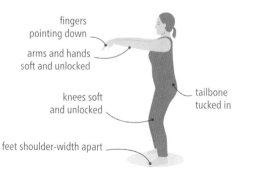

fingers pointing down

arms and hands soft and unlocked

knees soft and unlocked

tailbone tucked in

feet shoulder-width apart

CLEARING UNHELPFUL THOUGHTS

Flushing breath – two short inhales through the nose and one exhale swiftly through the mouth – can be used as a quick intervention to direct you away from unhelpful thoughts and behaviours. It also clears adrenaline from the system after a shock. Try this breath when you are meditating and it is challenging to sit still.

01

Choose a fixed point in front of you to "anchor" your gaze throughout the process. Start by taking 3–5 deep conscious breaths (see pages 18–19).

NEED TO KNOW

BENEFITS Relieves persistent thoughts, obsessional tendencies, and cravings; leaves you grounded, present, and empowered.

TIME Short bursts of 3–6 sets, but no more at a time.

focus on a fixed point ahead of you

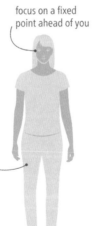

sit or stand somewhere you won't be disturbed

02

Take 2 audible, 1-second
in-breaths through the nose
in quick succession, making
the second one deeper
than the first.

03

Breathe an energized
2-second exhale through the
mouth. Picture the inhales
seeking and finding the
unwanted thoughts or
behaviours, and the exhales
flushing them out.

04

Repeat this sequence up
to 6 times, then pause and
see how you feel. Repeat up
to 6 more times if you feel
you need to. Afterwards,
go for a walk outdoors
if you can.

RETURNING TO FEELING

Diaphragmatic or belly breathing while cultivating a simple state of mindfulness will stimulate the neural networks between brain and body. This superhighway of nerves can be compromised when we suffer trauma, resulting in emotional numbness and reducing our sense of connection with others. See also pages 84–85, Breathing to Relieve Stress.

02

Start to extend the exhale so it is twice as long as the inhale (in for 2–4 seconds and out for 4–8). Breathe fully, opening up the diaphragm, and without moving your chest.

NEED TO KNOW

BENEFITS Increased sense of security, purpose, empathy, direction, and awareness.

TIME 5–10 minutes regularly through the day.

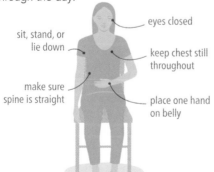

eyes closed

sit, stand, or lie down

keep chest still throughout

make sure spine is straight

place one hand on belly

01

Observe your breath then, breathing in and out slowly and deliberately through your nose, make your belly (not your chest) rise on the inhale and fall on the exhale for 3–5 breaths.

03

Keep this gentle cyclical breathing going and observe how your body feels. Notice any sensations that come to your attention and gently acknowledge them one by one.

04

After 5–10 minutes, start to normalize your breathing again, wiggle your fingers and toes, and open your eyes, coming back to awareness gently.

05

As an alternative, try breathing in through the nose and out through pursed lips as if through a straw. Try both methods and notice which feels better for you.

01

Choose a time and place where you will not be disturbed. Become aware of your breathing and notice how your body feels.

03

With the fingertips of one hand, gently stroke all over your other hand and forearm. Stroke very slowly, feeling with total mindful presence any specific sensations that arise.

02

Start a simple breath pattern such as conscious connected breathing (see pages 18–19) or ocean breath (see pages 36–37). Keep the breath soft and flowing.

CULTIVATING SELF CARE

Self-love can provide you with a much-yearned-for sense of wholeness and belonging. In its absence, we tend to seek it through attention from others or external activity, when in fact, we ourselves may be "the one" we've been waiting for. Regular practice of this exercise leaves you feeling replenished, resourced, and nurtured.

05

Do you feel softer
and more compassionate
or harder and more
armoured? Accept your
experience, however it
was for you.

04

Swap hands after 90 seconds
and, breathing continuously,
continue for 90 seconds more.
Gradually refocus on your
breathing, open your eyes
and become aware of your
surroundings once more.

NEED TO KNOW

BENEFITS Self-
acceptance; fewer bad
habits; confidence;
self-belief; contentment.

TIME Up to 3 minutes; as
needed.

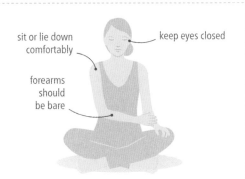

sit or lie down
comfortably

keep eyes closed

forearms
should
be bare

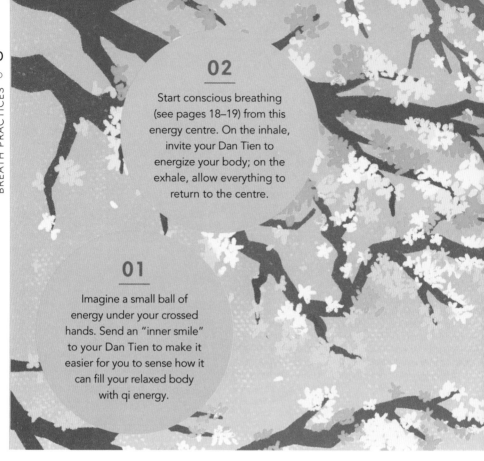

02

Start conscious breathing
(see pages 18–19) from this
energy centre. On the inhale,
invite your Dan Tien to
energize your body; on the
exhale, allow everything to
return to the centre.

01

Imagine a small ball of
energy under your crossed
hands. Send an "inner smile"
to your Dan Tien to make it
easier for you to sense how it
can fill your relaxed body
with qi energy.

BREATHING TO ACTIVATE
YOUR COMPASSION

According to the Dao Yin breath and movement practice
the lower Dan Tien, located just below your belly button, is
the qi energy centre of the body. Breathing to open it up
will reconnect you with your compassion, increase stamina,
willpower, and improve your general health.

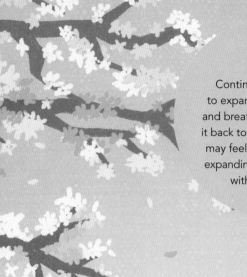

03

Continue breathing in
to expand your qi energy
and breathing out to return
it back to the Dan Tien. You
may feel your whole body
expanding and contracting
with the breath.

04

When you feel ready, take a
few longer breaths, extending
your exhales in particular to
return your energy to your
centre. Thank the energies you
have been working with,
then open your eyes.

NEED TO KNOW

BENEFITS Focus, energy,
or willpower; leaves you
grounded, vibrant, strong,
stable, and healthy.

TIME 3 minutes, or as long
as you can maintain your
conscious presence.

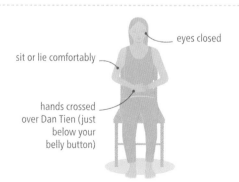

eyes closed

sit or lie comfortably

hands crossed
over Dan Tien (just
below your
belly button)

FINDING YOUR ROOTS

Although we all inhabit a body, due to the focus we put on mental activities like thinking and problem solving, it is easy to feel disconnected from our own physical experience. This breath practice gets you right back down to earth, where you can regain a sense of safety and stability. Don't worry too much about counting your breaths; instead focus on what feels right.

02

Take 3–5 slow breaths in through your nose and out through your mouth, releasing them with a soft sigh. Notice your chest gently open with these breaths.

NEED TO KNOW

BENEFITS Improves mental and physical stability, decisiveness; leaves you grounded.

TIME 3–5 minutes, or as long as needed.

eyes open, looking ahead

chin tilted slightly towards your chest

arms by your sides, palms facing forward

stand barefoot on the ground

01

Stand tall, preferably somewhere you have a view of nature. Fix your eyes on a point in the distance. Roll your shoulders back and release any tension you may be holding there.

03

Keep breathing in through the
nose and out through the mouth.
Take your awareness down your
body and release any tension
around your stomach/abdomen
area. Allow your stomach to feel
soft and full with no holding.

04

With the next few breaths,
take your awareness down to the
pelvis. Connect with these powerful
balancing and supportive bones.
Imagine your "roots" going down
into the earth and supporting you
completely. Be aware of being
rooted through your
legs and feet.

05

When you feel grounded
in your body, enjoy the
sensation of breathing
normally. Take your time
before closing the practice
with a gesture of completion
(see page 15).

01

In a park or garden where you will not be disturbed, choose a young tree to connect with. Stand, barefoot, a short distance from the tree's canopy.

03

Relax your arms down and, holding your palms open to the tree, use them to sense the energetic presence of the tree. With your next inhale, lift your arms up to the sky.

02

Breathing through your nose, stand with your palms together. Notice your breath and keep it flowing. Open your eyes and step towards the tree.

ALLEVIATING DEPRESSION

Breathing with awareness and spending time in nature are proven to help the symptoms of depression and reduce the need for medication. This ancient qigong practice sets up a circuit with energy flowing between a tree and ourselves. It reminds us that we are part of the natural world, and that time spent in nature can help us back into balance.

05

Repeat steps 3–4, drawing energy from the ground with the in-breath and returning it to the tree with the out-breath. After 20 repetitions, finish with a grateful bow to the tree and the earth.

04

Imagine your breath drawing the earth's energy up through your body to connect with the tree above you. Breathe out through your mouth, lowering your arms and imagining the energy travelling back down through the tree to the ground.

NEED TO KNOW

BENEFITS Optimism, hope, increased energy, creativity, and enthusiasm.

TIME Ongoing medium- to long-term practice; daily as necessary.

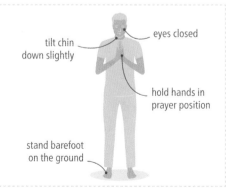

tilt chin down slightly

eyes closed

hold hands in prayer position

stand barefoot on the ground

OVERCOMING YOUR FEARS

Taking 20 connected nose breaths is a gentle process that helps to restore harmony to the body and mind by creating a space between you and feelings of uncertainty, insecurity, and panic. You imagine yourself breathing out fear and anxiety and breathing in peace and safety, which moves you beyond a pattern of negative thoughts and draining feelings.

02

Breathing through the nose, connect your inhale to your exhale with no gap. Take 4 breaths, then make the fifth longer and more exaggerated. This completes one set.

01

Decide how strong the fear sensation is in your body at this moment on a scale of 1–10, where 1 is hardly causing a problem and 10 is highly problematic.

NEED TO KNOW

BENEFITS Liberation; confidence; centred energy; focused thought; mental clarity; rejuvenation; a sense of personal empowerment.

TIME 1–3 minutes; several times a day as needed.

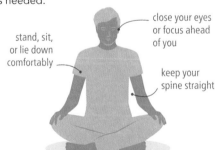

stand, sit, or lie down comfortably

close your eyes or focus ahead of you

keep your spine straight

03

Repeat this set of 5 breaths 3 more times to make 20 connected breaths in all. Use the fingers of your hands to help you keep count.

04

When you have completed a 20-breath cycle, assess how you feel and rate the fear sensation again. If the fear still feels strong, complete another cycle.

05

Keep breathing in this way until the fear feels more manageable. When you are ready, let your breathing return to normal.

BUILDING SELF-ESTEEM

This conscious, connected mouth-breathing exercise is a quick way to access your solar plexus, the internal "sun centre" of the body and its associated energies: confidence, assertiveness, autonomy, and willpower. It will boost your drive and passion for life, countering any day-to-day ill-effects of low self-worth.

02

As you exhale, allow your body to sink down onto the ball. Breathe in, noticing the pressure of your ribcage squeezing the ball.

NEED TO KNOW

BENEFITS Increased self-belief, drive, ambition, vision, and clarity.

TIME Daily practice; as needed.

EQUIPMENT Small soft stress ball (or rolled-up pair of socks).

start lying comfortably on your back

arms straight at your sides, palms up

place a stress ball under middle of your back

01

Become aware of your breathing. Relax your jaw and allow your mouth to drop open, which will open your throat. Breathe softly at your own pace in and out through your mouth.

03

As you breathe out, make an audible sigh. Experiment with noises that feel liberating to you. Breathe out any feelings of embarrassment or inhibition, embracing your power through sound.

04

After 3–5 minutes, remove the ball, roll onto your belly, and place the ball at the base of your sternum underneath your body, above your belly button. Rest your forehead on your hands.

05

Allow your weight to sink down, and again breathe into the pressure caused by the ball. For 3–5 minutes, use the in-breath to press the ball into the floor, and make a sound as you exhale. Breathe normally again and sit up gently.

SPEAKING YOUR TRUTH

Regular conscious breathing with sound helps build confidence in vocal self-expression. Finding words, and the confidence to express them, can be a challenge and trouble doing so may indicate that energy is blocked around the throat, the source of verbal communication. Try to reverberate the sound from as low down your body as you can, and not only from the throat.

01

Find a private spot and start conscious connected mouth breathing (see pages 18–19). Take a deep breath into your lower abdomen and release it while intoning "Aaaaay" (as in "hay").

NEED TO KNOW

BENEFITS Throat open and relaxed; easier self-expression; able to express and share thoughts or feelings.

TIME 5–10 mins; as long as needed.

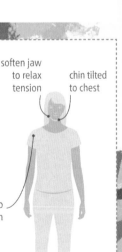

soften jaw to relax tension

chin tilted to chest

shoulders rolled back to ensure upper body open

stand comfortably

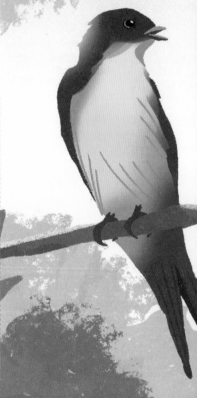

02

Exhale for as long as possible without pushing. Take 4 more breaths, and with each exhale make a different vowel sound: "Eeeee" (as in "key"); "Ayyye" (as in "hi"); "Ohhhhhh" (as in "slow"); and finally exhale to the sound of "Yuuuuu".

03

Still breathing consciously, say simple words or phrases confidently, for example "Yes!" or "No!" Do a few rounds of each before moving to the next word. Lower your pitch if the sound feels weak.

04

Sing, say, or breathe an affirmation such as "I am ready to open up full and authentic expression of my truth," "I am ready to feel heard," or "My voice is pleasing to me and those around me."

05

When you feel the exercise is complete, close with a simple gesture of completion (see page 15).

RELEASING ANGER

Although anger can be damaging when not expressed responsibly, its positive aspects keep us motivated, passionate, and productive. Trying to shut it down can be problematic, as pent-up emotion is bad for our physical health. Whenever you feel overwhelmed with anger, use this simple breathing exercise to safely access and release your inner "fire energy" and return to a grounded, relaxed state.

NEED TO KNOW

BENEFITS Balance; energy; focus; clarity; drive, determination, and ambition.

TIME 10–15 minutes, or as long as needed; may take several sessions.

use a mirror to gaze at your left eye

if necessary, massage your jaw to release it

tilt chin down, open mouth wide, and breathe through it

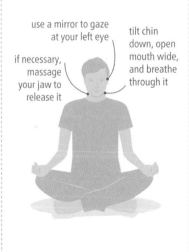

01

In a quiet, private place, begin to breathe deeply in a connected rhythm. Exaggerate the exhale, making a slight "Ha!" sound. Think of a cause of annoyance in your life.

02

Let yourself feel the emotion, then "flush" the anger out in the exhale. You can express your feelings out loud on the exhale, if you want to. If you begin to feel stressed, change to a gentle nose breath, keeping eye-contact in the mirror.

03

After a while you should feel that the emotion has moved on from your body. Return to breathing normally and bring your hands together to complete the session.

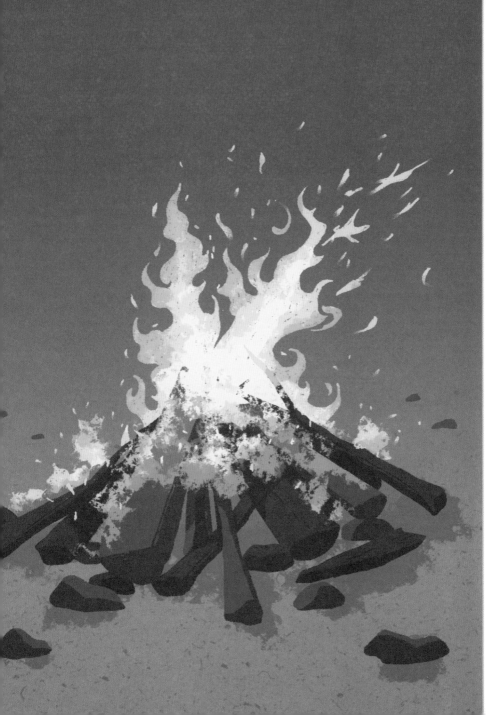

RELEASING JUDGMENT

This integrative breath process focuses on consciously breathing negative energy out of our bodies. It supports us to grow beyond habitual judgments, guilt, and shame. Repeated over time, it will help you become oriented towards positive, encouraging possibilities and away from blame, self-deprecation, and critical thoughts.

NEED TO KNOW

BENEFITS Liberation from judgment against yourself and others; flexibility.

TIME As long as necessary.

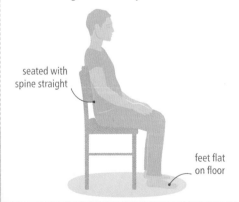

seated with spine straight

feet flat on floor

01

When a feeling of judgment arises, sit comfortably, take a few conscious connected breaths (see pages 18–19) and start to connect with your body.

02

Notice places where your body feels tight or pinched and direct your breath into that place. Expand the sensation with fuller breaths.

03

Breathe loving acceptance into that place. Ask yourself what that part of your body would say if it had a voice. Allow it to "speak", saying out loud the thoughts that come into your head.

04

Keep breathing consciously and continually, with the intention of releasing what is no longer needed as you exhale. Sensations may intensify or dissolve. Either is fine – accept where you are.

05

Finish by saying out loud: "The thought or judgment that has been holding me back is…" Take a breath and let it go, saying "I choose to rise above this belief to a time and place I feel free."

06

Take a big breath in and out to release the experience from your body. Repeat the process a few times until the judgmental feelings have softened in both your body and mind.

02

When the feeling starts to surface, use soft and rapid little sniffy breaths in and out through the nose to encourage the crying to open up. Resist the urge to tense up.

01

Find somewhere private and start conscious connected breathing (see pages 18–19) through the nose. Start to think about things that make you feel sad, using music or a film if it helps.

SURRENDERING TO TEARS

Studies show that a good cry really can improve your mood. Stress chemicals in your brain literally flow out in your tears, thereby alleviating sad feelings. Stifling emotional tears is linked to a higher risk of heart disease and hypertension. When emotion needs to leave your body, use conscious breathing to access your suppressed feelings.

03

Keep your breath light and allow your feelings to move through you. Try not to get stuck in a loop, and if you lose your breath connection, come back to breathing with awareness as soon possible.

04

When you come to a natural close, bring your hands to prayer in front of your heart as a gesture of gratitude. Close your eyes for a moment, then get on with your day.

NEED TO KNOW

BENEFITS Increased sense of lightness; relief; clarity; sensation of openness in chest.

TIME 10–15 minutes or as long as needed.

EQUIPMENT If needed, music or a film to activate sadness.

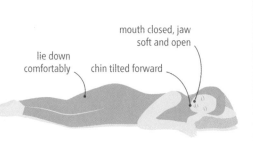

mouth closed, jaw soft and open

lie down comfortably

chin tilted forward

OVERCOMING CRAVINGS

When trying to leave a self-destructive habit behind, use your breath to redirect your mind from thoughts or behaviours that activate feelings of boredom, low self-worth, or lack of willpower. Long-term, consider seeking the support of a group or mentor to help you to stay strong in moments of weakness.

NEED TO KNOW

BENEFITS Mental clarity; freedom from compulsive and self-destructive thoughts; self-discipline.

TIME 5–10 mins; as long as needed.

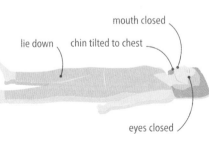

mouth closed

lie down   chin tilted to chest

eyes closed

02

When you feel comfortable belly-breathing, gently flex the muscles of your right foot and hold this tension for 20 breaths in and out.

01

Become aware of your breathing. With minimal chest-inhalation, breathe deeply in and out through your nose directly into your belly.

03

Let the muscles go, noting the sense of release as you do, and repeat with your left foot. Then repeat step 2 for both calves, thighs, arms, hands, and shoulders, tensing for 20 breaths each.

04

Complete the process with the muscles in your jaw, chin, and forehead. Maintain the deep belly-breathing through the exercise.

05

When you have finished, you might notice a warm, weightless feeling. Remain lying down in this relaxed state for as long as you wish, then get up and go for a walk if you can.

CULTIVATING INTIMACY

Eye-gazing is a simple way to deepen an intimate emotional connection, without the need for words. It is particularly helpful when we feel out of connection with our loved ones and talking seems to drive us further apart. Undertaken while breathing consciously, it allows us to meet each other afresh in the present moment.

01

Take a moment to settle into your bodies by closing your eyes and taking 3–5 deep conscious breaths (see pages 18–19).

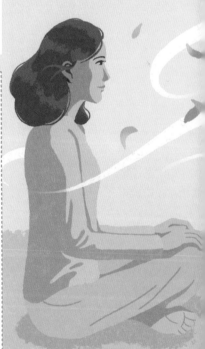

NEED TO KNOW

BENEFITS Heals a sense of separation; resolves relationship issues and conflict; fosters intimacy and trust.

TIME 10–30 minutes.

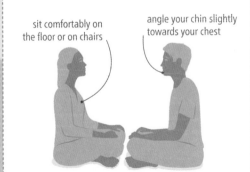

sit comfortably on the floor or on chairs

angle your chin slightly towards your chest

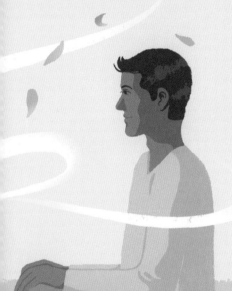

02

When you both feel ready, focus your attention on your partner's left eye. Soften your gaze, as if appreciating a beautiful scene in nature. Bring your attention to your breathing.

03

Breathe seamlessly, either in and out through the mouth, or in and out through the nose, keeping the inhale connected to the exhale with no pauses.

04

As you maintain eye contact, your perception of the person in front of you may change moment to moment. Allow these changes to pass without judgment.

05

Match your partner's breath pattern, timing your inhale and exhale to theirs. Notice how that feels. Continue in this way until you both reach a natural point of completion. Close with a gesture of completion, such as a hug.

BREATHING FOR PATIENCE

Use this controlled nose-breathing practice to regain emotional balance when you feel stressed about punctuality, whether waiting for someone or running late yourself. This kind of day-to-day stress with time-keeping can cause your body to release so-called "fight or flight" hormones which, if it happens too regularly, can cause health problems.

01

Support your back against a wall if you are standing, or lean into the back of your chair. Close your eyes or gaze at a fixed point ahead of you. Become aware of your breathing.

NEED TO KNOW

BENEFITS Reconnection to self and others; physical and psychological calm.

TIME 3–5 minutes.

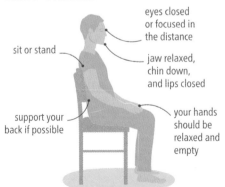

sit or stand

eyes closed or focused in the distance

jaw relaxed, chin down, and lips closed

support your back if possible

your hands should be relaxed and empty

02

Start by breathing in through your nose for the count of 2 and out for the count of 2. Repeat twice more to make a complete set of 3 breaths. Allow your breath to extend right into your belly.

03

Then for the next cycle, inhale for the count of 2 and out for 3. Repeat twice more. Then, for each new set of 3 breaths, allow 1 more count on the exhale, up to a count of 10 on the exhale.

04

When you reach 3 breaths exhaling to the count of 10, start to reverse the process by shortening your out-breath back to 9, 8, and so on all the way back to 3 breaths in and out to the count of 2. Release breath control.

05

Take 3 full relaxed breaths slowly in and out through your mouth and then return to normal breathing. You are now ready to get on with your day.

RELIEVING STEESS

When you feel your stress levels escalating, breathing out through pursed lips returns the breathing to a stable, healthy rhythm. Stress induces tension in the muscles, adversely affecting your internal organs and compromising your immune system. Long exhales are the quickest way to induce calm; use this technique to avoid a full-scale panic attack.

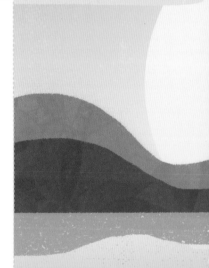

01

Become aware of your breath. Take a few natural breaths and soften and relax your body. Inhale slowly and deliberately through your nose for a count of 3–5 seconds.

NEED TO KNOW

BENEFITS Physically and psychologically more secure and stable; more grounded.

TIME As needed; ongoing daily practice.

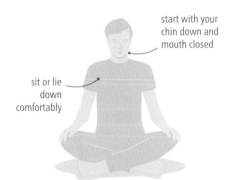

start with your chin down and mouth closed

sit or lie down comfortably

02

Purse your lips as if you were about to whistle. Breathe out slowly through your pursed lips, exhaling without straining, for about twice as long as your inhale.

03

Continue to breathe in through your nose and slowly out through your pursed lips, directing your breath to fill your belly, not your chest.

04

Keep this breathing going for as long as it feels helpful for you. When you are ready to stop, move slowly and deliberately, awakening your body by wiggling your fingers and toes.

SPIRITUAL SELF

For thousands of years, mystics and devotees have used breath control to access non-ordinary states of consciousness. Breathwork is now being rediscovered as a safe and effective way to journey into the subconscious to experience the wonder and revelations of our inner world.

INTEGRATING MIND, BODY, AND SPIRIT

This exercise teaches holographic breathing, where you breathe through your nose while your lips are closed and the tongue is on the roof of your mouth. At the same time, the jaw gently opens on the in-breath and closes on the out. This brings a deep sense of relaxation and meditation and can open up spiritual insights.

01

Breathing through your nose, and with the lips closed, bring the upper surface of your tongue to the roof of your mouth. Do this through the whole meditation.

NEED TO KNOW

BENEFITS A feeling of harmony and balance; sense of connectivity, purpose, and clarity.

TIME Start with 10 minutes and increase over time.

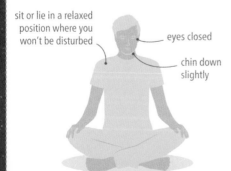

sit or lie in a relaxed position where you won't be disturbed

eyes closed

chin down slightly

02

Keeping the lips closed, start making a relaxed up-and-down movement of the jaw, almost as if you were chewing. This jaw movement is small, only about half-a-finger width.

03

Now, slow the movement down and as your jaw opens, let the breath come in through your nose, and as it closes, let the breath come out through your nose. Remember to keep your lips closed and tongue on the roof of the mouth.

04

When you feel ready, shift so the emphasis is on the breath first. As you breathe in through the nose, let the jaw relax open; as you breathe out, let the jaw relax closed. Allow yourself to relax into this.

05

On the out breath, allow the teeth to touch lightly or not at all. After a while, allow the whole body to breathe and let the jaw follow. When you are ready, slowly come back to awareness.

DEVELOPING PSYCHIC SKILLS

Intuition and psychic abilities often come from our connection with nature and the higher energies. Holographic breathing allows you to connect more fully with these realms, with a subtle breathing motion through your body and head. You can use this meditation to develop the sensitivity needed for intuitive insight.

02

Also notice whether you can feel a subtle opening and closing through the face and head with the breath. If you can, spend some time with this.

NEED TO KNOW

BENEFITS Boosts empathic capabilities; increased sensitivity, insight, and intuition.

TIME Start with 5-10 minutes and increase over time.

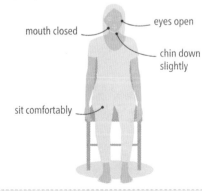

eyes open

mouth closed

chin down slightly

sit comfortably

01

Gently start holographic breathing (see page 88). Feel the breath opening and closing through your whole body and feel the jaw gently moving, too.

03

Now feel this motion of the breath through the whole body, including arms, legs, face, and head. Everywhere is opening on the in-breath and closing on the out-breath. Notice the jaw following along. Spend time with this.

04

Notice if you can feel the earth breathing with you in its own way and that the universe and higher energies are also breathing. Spend some time breathing and connecting with them all.

05

When you feel ready to close, thank the earth and higher energies, breathe gently for a while then let yourself come back.

HEALING SEPARATION

One of the more complex sensations of the human psyche is a deep sense of separation, which can be a result of physical or emotional distance, or internal conflict. This exercise uses conscious breathing with a technique called parts integration, from Neuro-linguistic Programming therapy. It can be very useful to harmonize your internal or external divisions.

02

Keeping your breath rhythmic, gentle, and connected, hold a hand palm-up and invite one of the parts to occupy it. Invite the other part into your opposite hand.

NEED TO KNOW

BENEFITS Increased integration and harmony with others; a feeling of connectivity and acceptance.

TIME 5–10 minutes.

01

Connect with your breathing, and shift into gentle conscious connected breathing (see pages 18–19) through the nose. Focus on the two parts involved in your sense of separation.

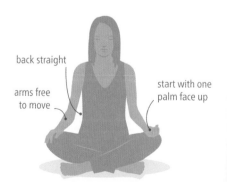

back straight

arms free
to move

start with one
palm face up

03

Remind yourself the purpose
is to bring these separated parts
together. Without moving your
arms, turn your palms to face
each other. With 3–5 conscious
breaths per hand, send love
and acknowledgment for
each part.

04

Take a deeper in-breath
and start to move your hands
together, letting go of any
resistance or tension on your
out-breath. Imagine the sides
begin to merge as you close
the gap between them.

05

When you feel ready,
draw both hands to your heart.
Notice how it feels to have fully
accepted both parts. Take a
deeper breath and close with
a gesture of completion
and balance.

ATTRACTING YOUR TRIBE

Whether you call it "conscious community" or "tribe", a sense of mutual connection and cooperation with the people in your life is highly desirable. This is a breath visualization to help you attract those who are able to love and support you in your development and growth. Breathe in to make yourself receptive and breathe out what you no longer need.

NEED TO KNOW

BENEFITS Sharing, exchanging, inspiring, and cross-pollinating with kindred spirits.

TIME 5–10 minutes; daily; on-going.

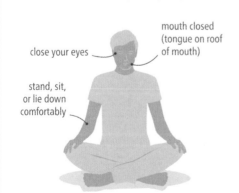

close your eyes

mouth closed (tongue on roof of mouth)

stand, sit, or lie down comfortably

01

Take a few deep conscious breaths (see pages 18–19). On an in-breath, imagine a spark of colourful light igniting in your belly and becoming brighter with each breath.

05

When you are ready, gently come back to your body. Steeple your hands to close, and trust healing connections will now be on their way to you.

04

Use your breath to connect with this vision as deeply as you can. Energize this scene with your faith and conviction that what you are seeking is also seeking you, right now.

03

Continue to breathe consciously and picture the light travelling out of the building and rising into the sky. See your light join other lights and enjoy this sense of connection.

02

Deepen your normal breath, keeping it rhythmic and connected. Imagine the light continuing to get brighter and bigger with each breath, forming a balloon of light around you.

MARKING RITES OF PASSAGE

Many societies hold traditional rituals to mark the transition from childhood to adolescence. You can perform this shamanic breath practice ritual together to commemorate your child reaching their next life stage. Such rites of passage acknowledge and respect young people in their development, as they grow into their autonomy and personal power.

01

Breathing consciously (see pages 18–19) as you prepare, choose a context that suits you both. You can use music, or props such as a photos and mementos.

NEED TO KNOW

BENEFITS A sense of purpose, clarity, and belonging in the world.

TIME As long as you both wish; followed by a celebration to mark the occasion.

02

Sit, lie, or even walk comfortably together. Ask your child to breathe consciously, taking slow, distinctly audible, not passive breaths of equal length in and out.

choose any position and setting that suits you

mouth closed, breathing through nose

03

Recount the key events in your child's life so far – if it helps, prepare a short script to read. As you continue to breathe together, share your joy at having them in your life, and your excitment that they are ready for the next level.

04

Invite your child to imagine a doorway into this new world, and to step through and see what lies ahead. Remind your child that you will always be there, then slowly come back to the present with some deeper breaths.

05

When you are ready, come to a close by bringing your hands together in a prayer position, maintaining eye contact with each other. Then plan a celebration of this new stage together.

MEETING YOUR SPIRIT GUIDES

Use this breath visualization to help you when you are looking for direction and purpose or seeking spiritual insight. Using conscious breath, journey through the realms of your imagination to find a magical animal to guide you through life's challenges. This animal, with the power to protect and advise you, is your Spirit Guide.

01

Find a quiet spot and play a relaxing music track for 10–15 minutes. With eyes closed or covered, start conscious breathing (see pages 18–19) through your nose.

02

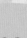

Put a hand on your belly to feel it rise and fall as you breathe in and out fully. Continuing to breathe in this way, imagine yourself on a path through a forest.

NEED TO KNOW

BENEFITS Sense of connectivity; quiet grounded presence.

TIME 10–20 minutes; repeat when guidance is needed; can be done along with Marking Rites of Passage (see pages 96–97).

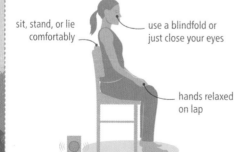

sit, stand, or lie comfortably

use a blindfold or just close your eyes

hands relaxed on lap

03

Gradually become aware of
your imagined surroundings
– are you in a forest? In the
mountains or on the coast?
Breathe to get a clear sense of
the landscape. Follow your
path to reach a clearing.

04

Once there, do you sense
another being? An instantly
recognizable creature, or one
that takes a while to emerge?
Keep your breath moving until
you glimpse your animal
guide. Let them approach.

05

Become aware of the
animal's characteristics and
how they might support you.
Breathe for a while with them,
then thank them and agree to
stay connected. Gradually come
back to the here-and-now by
taking deep breaths.

CREATING YOUR REALITY

At times of confusion, use this simple exercise to clear your head and provide clarity for your next steps in life. Derived from the yogic Walking the Eight active breathwork meditation, the exercise involves walking in a figure-of-eight while breathing with awareness to balance the hemispheres of your brain. The more you practise, the more profound the exercise becomes.

NEED TO KNOW

BENEFITS Calmness; clarity; direction; insight; awareness.

TIME 15 minutes or as long as needed; daily.

EQUIPMENT Two stones or other objects to make islands on the ground.

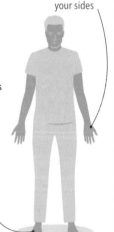

hands loose by your sides

barefoot if possible

01

Find a large enough, level space inside or out, where you won't be disturbed. Place 2 stones far enough apart for you to walk a figure of 8 around them comfortably.

02

Stand between the stones. Close your eyes and start conscious connected breathing (see pages 18–19) through your nose to your belly, feeling it soften.

03

When you feel ready,
open your eyes and start to walk
clockwise in a figure of 8 at your
own pace, circling first one stone
and then the other. Breathe
continuously; the deeper you
breathe, the more profound
the experience.

04

Keep walking and breathing
for about 15 minutes, allowing
thoughts and feelings to come
and go. You can vary your pace or
pause at the centre. With practice,
you will be able to lift your eyes
from the ground as you walk.

05

To complete, slow
down and stop halfway
between the stones. Finish
with your hands in the
prayer position, in a gesture
of gratitude.

02

Extend the in-breath down
into your belly and then up
through your diaphragm to
gently fill your chest. Balance
the inhale and the exhale. On
the next exhale, release any
tension in your body.

01

Close your eyes and
sink into your body, taking
3–5 deep breaths through
your nose. Start conscious
connected breathing
(see pages 18–19).

BREATHING FOR PEACE

Use this meditative exercise whenever you need to restore
your inner peace. Visualizing a peaceful image while
breathing consciously will transport you into a harmonious
realm, helping you find serenity in both your inner and outer
worlds – the world around you will reflect back your more
stabilized state, like a clear reflection in a still pond.

03

Keeping your breathing connected, invite an image you find peaceful and calming into your mind. Make the image as detailed as you can to experience the scene. Enjoy being there.

04

Notice how it feels to drop deeply into this imagined place. When you are ready, let the image fade, exhale a wave of peaceful energy out into the world, and return to your day.

NEED TO KNOW

BENEFITS Tranquility; acceptance; understanding; empowerment.

TIME 5 minutes.

lie in any comfortable position with your body open and relaxed

close your eyes

play relaxing music

HARMONIZING YOUR MALE AND FEMALE ENERGY

In the Hindu and Taoist traditions, we all have two energy fields within us – feminine (yin: creative and receptive) and masculine (yang: active and driven). An imbalance of the two can adversely affect your mindset. Use this breath practice, with its active inhale and passive exhale, to cultivate a "Union of Opposites" inside you.

02

Pause at the top of the inhale, then gently exhale, noticing the sense of letting go and releasing. Pause before taking the next breath.

01

Start conscious connected nose-breathing (see pages 18–19). Then take a longer, stronger breath and bring your full attention to it.

NEED TO KNOW

BENEFITS Integrates giving and receiving; cultivates sensitivity.

TIME 10–15 minutes daily.

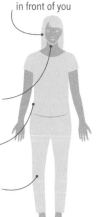

eyes closed or focused in front of you

mouth closed, breathing through your nose throughout

straight spine

stand, sit, or lie where you won't be disturbed

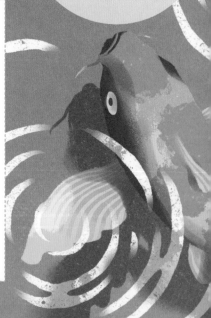

03

Breathe in again when you feel the impulse, noticing how it feels. Continue breathing this way. Observe whether the inhale, exhale, or pause between breaths feels most comfortable.

04

When you are ready, lift your hands into the prayer position on an inhale. As you exhale, let your hands return to their original position. Inhaling, lift your hands; exhaling, release them.

05

Bring your hands up for a final time as a gesture of completion, closure, and balance. Take a few breaths in and out before releasing your hands one last time.

BREATHWORK INTERVENTIONS

This section provides you with a set of tools for your breathwork "first-aid" box. Practise them when you feel relaxed and grounded, so that if you need any of them in a moment of discomfort or crisis, they will be familiar and easy to recall.

01

Lying comfortably or sitting, start holographic breathing (see pages 88–89). Bring your awareness to your chest and abdomen.

03

Notice that it feels as if your whole body, including the jaw, is opening on the in-breath, and closing on the out-breath. Breathe like this in a gentle way for a while. Become aware of the area around the pain, and also allow this to breathe.

02

As the chest and abdomen expand with your in-breath, the jaw gently opens, and as they close with your out-breath, the jaw closes. Become aware of your whole body including your arms, legs, and head.

BREATHING THROUGH PAIN

Holographic breathing helps bring relaxation and the subtle motion of the breath to areas of pain or illness, which can help with distressing symptoms and aid recovery. You can also use this exercise to bring self care or wellness to any part of your body.

05

Breathe and relax through your whole body. Become aware that everything is connected and gently breathing together, including the painful area. When you are ready, gently allow yourself to come back.

04

Now include the area where you feel pain, letting it breathe with the whole body in a very gentle way. Allow this whole area to relax with the gentle motion of the breath, and imagine wellbeing going to this area.

NEED TO KNOW

BENEFITS Symptom relief; a sense of wholeness and wellbeing.

TIME 5–10 minutes; repeat as needed.

lie or sit comfortably

eyes closed

keep lips closed

01

Still all movement in
your body, as activity can
contribute to disorientation.
Close your mouth and breathe
in and out through your
nose. Place one hand
on your belly.

02

With the thumb of your free
hand, close one nostril and
breathe in slowly through the
other. Inflate your lungs as much
as possible – your in-breath
should lift your belly hand
slightly.

COUNTERING DIZZINESS

This exercise helps you to overcome any dizziness
caused by a disruption in the balance of oxygen and carbon
dioxide resulting from shallow, rapid chest breaths. Known
as Back-to-Earth breathing, it regulates and deepens your
breath pattern to restore balance. Seek professional help if
you experience persistent dizziness without known cause.

03

At the top of the in-breath, hold your breath for a second and purse your lips as if to whistle. Let the air out slowly to a count of 5 through your pursed lips, emptying your lungs as much as possible.

05

Repeat the cycle 5 times for each nostril (more if needed) then return to breathing normally. Take your time standing up, with slow movements.

04

Notice how your belly hand drops again as you breathe out. Apply a little pressure if that helps with a fuller exhale. This completes 1 cycle.

NEED TO KNOW

BENEFITS Increased sense of safety; stability; calm; groundedness.

TIME 1–3 minutes; as needed.

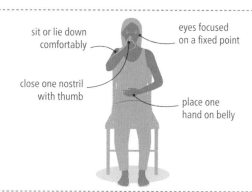

sit or lie down comfortably

eyes focused on a fixed point

close one nostril with thumb

place one hand on belly

BREATHING BEYOND NAUSEA

Anyone who has experienced morning-sickness, motion-sickness, or a stomach bug knows how debilitating these can be. Whether the source of your nausea is physical or psychological, focusing on deep, controlled breathing has been proven in clinical trials to reduce the severity of the symptoms. Do this exercise to help you feel grounded again.

02

Take a normal breath in and out through your nose, followed by a deeper, slower breath, again through your nose.

NEED TO KNOW

BENEFITS Soothing for the stomach; relaxing for the mind.

TIME As long and as regularly as needed.

CAUTION Seek medical help for persistent nausea.

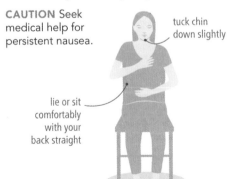

tuck chin down slightly

lie or sit comfortably with your back straight

01

Bring stillness to your body in a comfortable seated or lying position, with your eyes closed or focused on a fixed point. Lightly place one hand on your belly and the other on your chest.

03

Let your chest and belly expand fully on the deep inhale and contract fully on the exhale. Notice your hands lift and drop with your breath. Keep taking a regular breath followed by a deeper breath.

04

As you breathe, imagine breathing the sick feeling out of your body. Picture a colour or shape where the sensation is most intense in your body. Allow that colour or shape to lift out of your body on the deep exhale.

05

Now allow a colour or image that brings you pleasure to come into your awareness. Use the deep inhale to breathe it into your body to replace the nausea. Continue for as long as you feel you need to.

BREATHING THROUGH SHOCK AND TRAUMA

When you experience a stressful event your body releases "fight or flight" hormones that can make you feel shaky, sweaty, and destabilized. If this happens to you, use this deep-breathing exercise to help you think more clearly, relieve muscle tension, and release unwanted stress.

01

Once the threat, trigger, or cause of upset has been dealt with, be still and bring your attention to your breath.

NEED TO KNOW

BENEFITS Increased sense of calm; groundedness, stability and clarity.

TIME As long as needed; use regularly to ease emotional stress.

02

Take a few deep breaths in and out through your nose. If your nose feels blocked, breathe in through your mouth, making a small "O" shape with your lips, as if sucking through a straw.

let the ground or a chair support you as you sit or lie down

eyes closed or focused in front of you

lie still, with hands unclenched

03
———

Now start to control
your breathing by slowly
inhaling, right down to your
belly. Hold the breath for a
moment, then exhale slowly
through your mouth.

04
———

Continuing this breath pattern,
focus on identifying 5 colours
around you; alternatively, close
your eyes and either notice the
noises you can hear or stroke
your forearm lightly with
your fingertips.

05
———

When you are ready, open
your eyes, gently shake your
hands and feet, and roll your
shoulders. Get a sense of
being safely in your body
before standing up.

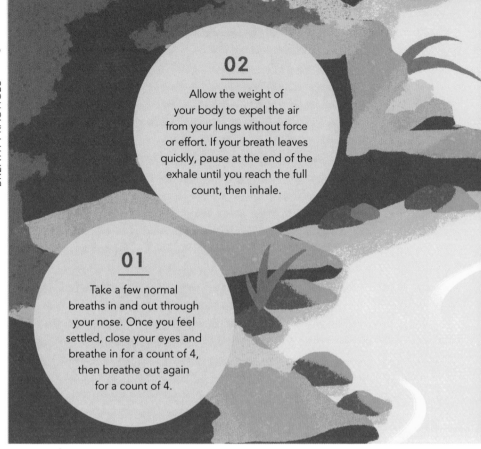

02

Allow the weight of
your body to expel the air
from your lungs without force
or effort. If your breath leaves
quickly, pause at the end of the
exhale until you reach the full
count, then inhale.

01

Take a few normal
breaths in and out through
your nose. Once you feel
settled, close your eyes and
breathe in for a count of 4,
then breathe out again
for a count of 4.

PREVENTING PALPITATIONS

When you feel your heart pounding, fluttering, or beating
irregularly, sometimes accompanied by sensations in your
throat or neck, use this integrative breathwork exercise to
get your body back into a natural rhythm and calm your
mind. This exercise is also useful when you feel stressed
or anxious, and to help you go to sleep.

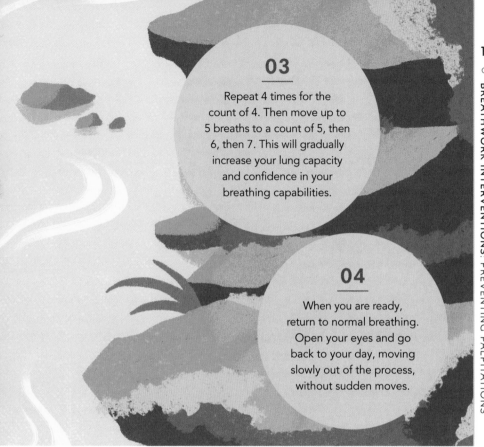

03

Repeat 4 times for the count of 4. Then move up to 5 breaths to a count of 5, then 6, then 7. This will gradually increase your lung capacity and confidence in your breathing capabilities.

04

When you are ready, return to normal breathing. Open your eyes and go back to your day, moving slowly out of the process, without sudden moves.

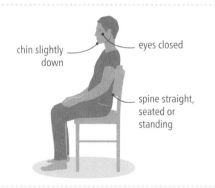

NEED TO KNOW

BENEFITS Reduction in symptoms; calmer; more grounded; more centred.

TIME 1–3 minutes; as needed; the more regular the better.

CAUTION Seek medical help if you experience dizziness, breathlessness, or chest pain.

chin slightly down

eyes closed

spine straight, seated or standing

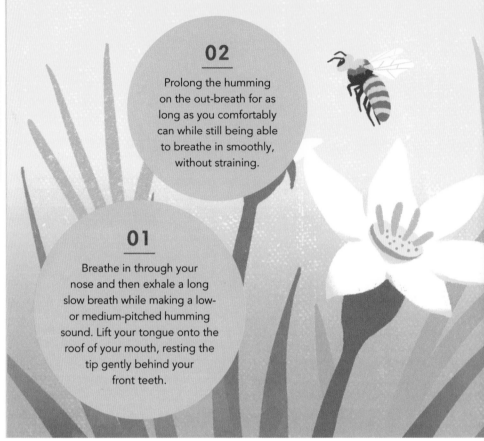

02

Prolong the humming on the out-breath for as long as you comfortably can while still being able to breathe in smoothly, without straining.

01

Breathe in through your nose and then exhale a long slow breath while making a low- or medium-pitched humming sound. Lift your tongue onto the roof of your mouth, resting the tip gently behind your front teeth.

RELIEVING HEADACHES

The Humming Bee Technique, a simple pranayama practice, uses the healing vibration of sound. Reverberations in the body can be directed to areas in need of support, and can help within just a few breaths. It is deeply therapeutic, partly since the long exhale calms the autonomic nervous system.

03

Feel how the sound waves gently vibrate your tongue, teeth, and sinuses. You may even notice a vibrational reverberation around your cranium, brain, and other parts of your body.

04

Repeat this practice for 6 rounds of breath. Then, keeping your eyes closed, return to your normal breathing. Notice anything different about your body: does it feel lighter or heavier, more open or more closed?

NEED TO KNOW

BENEFITS Improves concentration; relieves hypertension; prevents or relieves migraine or headache.

TIME 5 minutes, or as long as feels good; when you have a migraine or feel one starting.

mouth closed, jaw relaxed — eyes closed

chin slightly downturned

sit in a chair, feet flat, or sit comfortably on the floor

BREATHING FOR HIGH BLOOD PRESSURE

If your breathing is fast, shallow, or irregular, your under-functioning diaphragm can place a burden on your cardiovascular system, raising your blood pressure. Practise this Coherent Breathing® exercise regularly to encourage a slower, rhythmic deep-breathing pattern, which has been proven to reduce blood pressure and balance the cardiovascular system.

NEED TO KNOW

BENEFITS Improved health of internal organs; lower blood pressure; relaxation; increased sense of wellbeing.

TIME 20 minutes daily for 21 consecutive days.

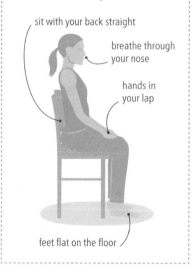

sit with your back straight

breathe through your nose

hands in your lap

feet flat on the floor

01

Synchronize your breathing at about 5 breaths per minute, making both the in- and out-breaths 6 seconds in length. A little longer or shorter is fine, but keep your breaths even.

02

Try to develop a deep letting-go sensation when you exhale. It's important to feel comfortable, so if you experience any physical discomfort, come back to normal breath before starting again.

03

Continue to breathe in this way for about 20 minutes. The eventual goal is to get into the habit of always breathing slowly, deeply, and rhythmically.

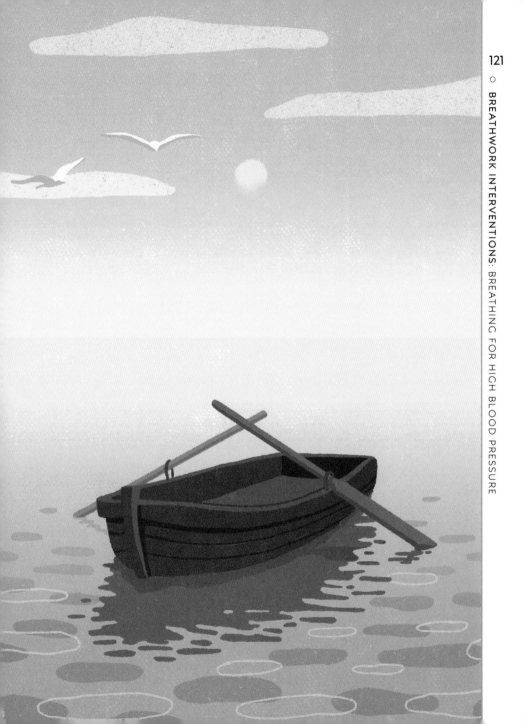

BREATHING TO RELIEVE ASTHMA

If you suffer from asthma you may breathe more quickly than most people. You're also likely to breathe through your mouth, exposing your lung tissue to dry, cool air, which can worsen your condition. Use this simple exercise to breathe calmly and slowly through your nose. Practised regularly, it will help you relax and may relieve your symptoms.

01

Sit comfortably and relax your body, focusing specifically on softening your belly and chest muscles. Allow your eyes to close and tilt your head slightly upward.

NEED TO KNOW

BENEFITS Increases breath confidence; can reduce use of inhalers.

TIME As long as needed to calm the breathing; regular daily practice.

CAUTION Talk to your GP before embarking on this exercise.

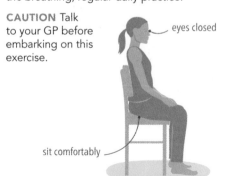

eyes closed

sit comfortably

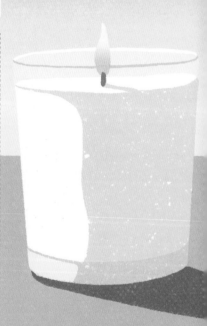

02

Now take a gentle, slow, shallow breath in through your nose while keeping your mouth closed. Breathe out slowly until you feel your lungs have been emptied of air.

03

Pause for as long as you can, then when you feel the urge, start the breathing cycle again. Repeat until your symptoms ease or you feel a sense of completion.

02

Contract your low belly,
pressing your hand to force
the breath out in a short burst.
Quickly release the contraction,
taking a short automatic and
passive in-breath; focus on
exhaling quickly, also
through the nose.

01

Bring your awareness
to your lower belly, and
place your hand on it.
Inhale deeply through
both nostrils.

CLEARING CONGESTION

This advanced pranayama exercise, known as Skull Shining
Breath, is effective at rejuvenating the internal organs. It
addresses many sub-ventilation issues caused by shallow
chest breathing. Short, powerful exhales and passive inhales
through the nose tone and cleanse the internal organs by
encouraging the cellular release of toxins.

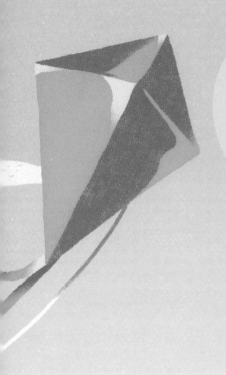

03

Continue breathing in
and out in this way, working
up to achieve 65–70 cycles in
a minute. With experience,
gradually quicken the pace,
increasing to 95–105 cycles
per minute.

04

After 1 minute of the
exercise, inhale deeply
through your nostrils, and
then exhale slowly through
your mouth to complete
the process. Stand
up slowly.

NEED TO KNOW

BENEFITS Invigoration; cleanses
respiratory system; and strengthens
diaphragm and abdominal muscles.

TIME Start with 10–20 seconds,
up to 1–3 minutes with practice.

CAUTION Do not do if you have high
blood pressure, heart disease, hernia,
respiratory disease, or are pregnant.

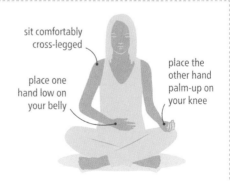

sit comfortably
cross-legged

place one
hand low on
your belly

place the
other hand
palm-up on
your knee

BREATHING THROUGH ANXIETY

This box-breathing exercise is a good all-rounder for regaining emotional and physical balance. Involving deep intentional breathing, it can lower your blood pressure and provide an immediate sense of calm, reducing stress and improving your mood and concentration. Teach the technique to youngsters who have difficulty regulating their moods and energy levels.

NEED TO KNOW

BENEFITS Relaxation; focus; sense of perspective.

TIME Repeat 4 times in 1 sitting; repeat several times a day to calm your nerves.

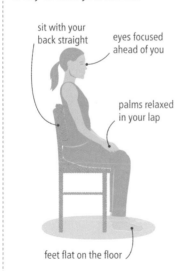

sit with your back straight

eyes focused ahead of you

palms relaxed in your lap

feet flat on the floor

01

Slowly empty your lungs through your mouth. Breathe in deeply through your nose to a slow count of 4, filling your lungs and then your abdomen. Avoid straining.

02

At the top of the inhale, hold your breath for a second slow count of 4. Now breathe out through your nose for another slow count of 4. Notice the air gently leaving your lungs. Then hold your breath for the same slow count of 4.

03

Repeat the process until you have done 4 box-breathing sets, then bring your hands into the prayer position in front of your heart as a gesture of closure.

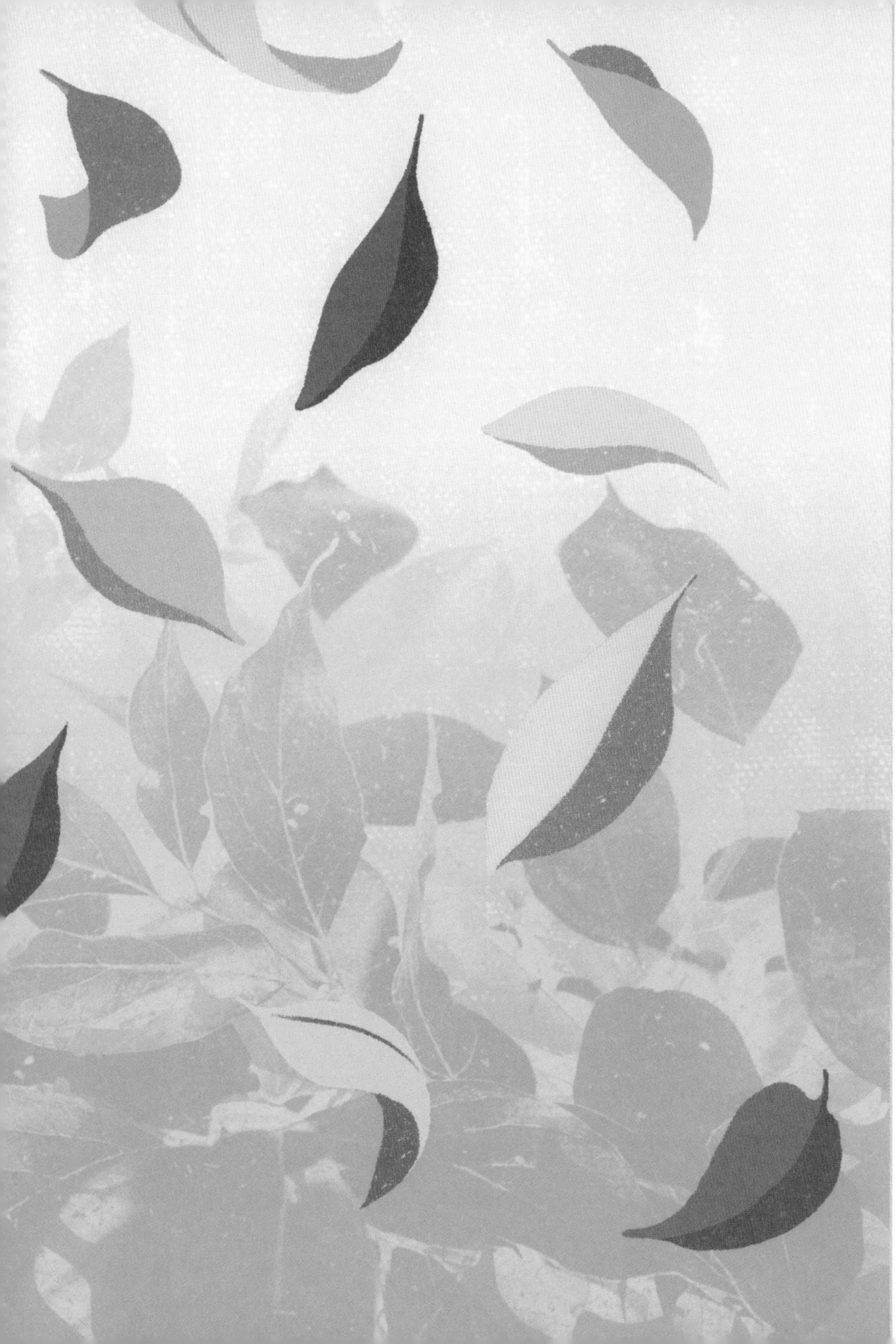

01

Gently inhale through your nose
into your belly for 4 seconds,
then release the breath through
pursed lips for 6 seconds. Use
the out-breath to allow any
tension to leave your body.

03

As you continue to breathe,
use powerful affirmations to
release any anxieties, guilt,
or shame you may feel about
your body and your
menstrual pain.

02

Keep this breath
pattern going, with your
breath reaching down to
your belly. It's important to
feel comfortable, so avoid
straining yourself in
any way.

BREATHING FOR
MENSTRUAL PAIN

If you suffer from menstrual pain, try this simple breathing process
to ease your symptoms. It works by extending the exhaled breath
to stimulate your body's soothing parasympathetic system. The
deep abdominal breathing gently massages the womb area
internally, increasing blood circulation and helping you relax.

05

When you feel ready,
bring your awareness back to
your abdomen area, sending
thanks to your womb. Bring your
hands into the prayer position as
a gesture of completion, open
your eyes, and gently get on
with your day.

04

Breathing in and out between
each phrase, say out loud "I love
and accept myself as a woman";
"My monthly cycle is natural and
healthy"; "I choose a pain-free
moon-cycle"; or other
affirmations of your own.

NEED TO KNOW

BENEFITS Soothes the
body; relaxes the mind.

TIME 2–3 minutes for as
long as needed.

CAUTION Seek medical
help for persistent nausea.

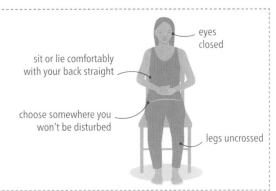

sit or lie comfortably
with your back straight

choose somewhere you
won't be disturbed

eyes
closed

legs uncrossed

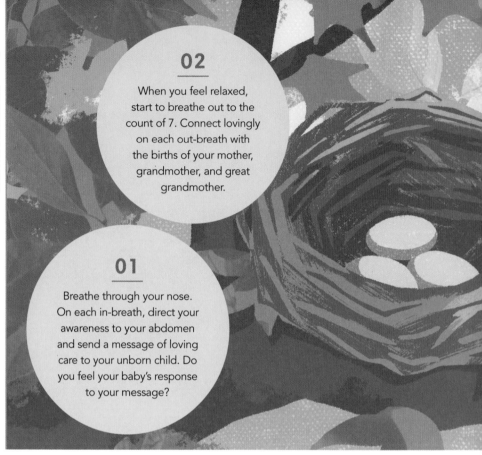

02

When you feel relaxed, start to breathe out to the count of 7. Connect lovingly on each out-breath with the births of your mother, grandmother, and great grandmother.

01

Breathe through your nose. On each in-breath, direct your awareness to your abdomen and send a message of loving care to your unborn child. Do you feel your baby's response to your message?

BREATHING DURING PREGNANCY

Pregnancy can be an anxious time. Practise this visualization exercise to help you connect positively with your unborn baby, with your own birth, and with those of your mother and your grandmother. Use your breath to release any negative emotions, doubts, and fears, layer by layer.

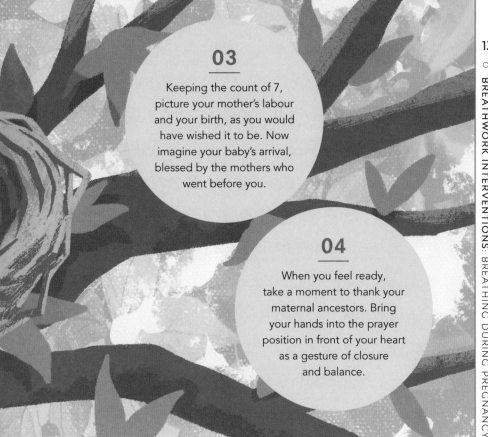

03

Keeping the count of 7, picture your mother's labour and your birth, as you would have wished it to be. Now imagine your baby's arrival, blessed by the mothers who went before you.

04

When you feel ready, take a moment to thank your maternal ancestors. Bring your hands into the prayer position in front of your heart as a gesture of closure and balance.

NEED TO KNOW

BENEFITS Increased comfort in your body; empowerment; trust in yourself.

TIME 15-minute breathing visualization; daily preparation for birth.

sit or lie down

choose somewhere you won't be disturbed

eyes closed or focused in front of you

01

Breathe in through your
nose and out through your
mouth, sighing or yawning to
open your jaw fully, but
without straining. Your inhale
should be slightly shorter
than your exhale.

03

As you breathe, notice that
your body is a safe place to be.
If you feel inspired, say out loud
"My body is safe" or "I feel safe
in my body right now". Imagine
you, your mother, and your
grandmother, all experiencing
beautiful births.

02

Relax your throat and start making
low vibrating sounds on each
out-breath. Your jaw and throat
are connected to your sexual
centre, so this will encourage your
pelvic region to relax. Move any
other parts of your body if you
feel the urge to.

BREATHING FOR BIRTH

If you're about to give birth, you can use this conscious
breathing exercise to help alleviate any fears you may have
about the birth process or doubts about your ability to manage
the strong sensations of labour. Your unborn baby can also
benefit from your positive shift in energy as you surrender to
your breath and embrace the birth, trusting that all will be well.

05

When you are ready, take a moment to thank your mother's line. Allow your breathing to return to normal and place your hands on your abdomen. Thank your little one for coming to you, so you can share this exciting journey.

04

Keep breathing out any anxieties or fears. Continue inviting your body to relax and open itself to sound, movement, and breath. Finally, imagine your precious baby's birth – smooth and delightful, and blessed by your ancestors.

NEED TO KNOW

BENEFITS Encourages trust; allows the birth process to progress to the next level.

TIME As long as needed.

CAUTION Seek medical help for persistent nausea.

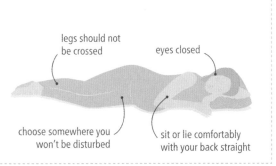

legs should not be crossed

eyes closed

choose somewhere you won't be disturbed

sit or lie comfortably with your back straight

BREATHING TO COOL DOWN

This pranayama practice known as Cooling Breath is perfect when you are feeling over-heated due to hot weather or following intensive exercise. If you struggle to curl your tongue into the recommended "U" shape (not everyone is able to), simply bend the sides up as much as you comfortably can and make an "O" shape with your lips.

01

Relax your jaw and your tongue and let your mouth drop open slightly. Roll your tongue into a "U" shape, poking the tip of your tongue just outside of your lips.

NEED TO KNOW

BENEFITS Feeling cooler; temperature regulation; calmer disposition; clearer outlook.

TIME 3 minutes, or longer if needed to cool down.

eyes closed

jaw relaxed and mouth dropped open a little

first finger and thumb touching, hands on knees

02

Inhale deeply through your rolled tongue and mouth. Imagine your tongue as a drinking straw, and that you are dragging cooling air up into the straw.

03

You may notice a cooling sensation as the air moves across the surface of your tongue. Breathe fully into your abdomen and then exhale fully through your nose.

04

Repeat this cycle for approximately 3 minutes, or as long as feels comfortable for you. To close, on the last inhale, retain your breath for a few seconds. Exhale and relax.

BREATHING FOR ALLERGY RELIEF

Bellows breath is an effective and dynamic pranayama breathing technique, which oxygenates your body and clears nasal congestion, alleviating allergy symptoms. The practice involves the abdomen moving rapidly during exhalation and inhalation, which stimulates the digestive tract and encourages the elimination of waste.

02

If your nose is very blocked, start gently. If not, aim to inhale and exhale more forcefully, making your belly move rapidly in and out.

NEED TO KNOW

BENEFITS Clear nasal passages; improved immune system; purified blood.

TIME 3 x sets of 10 breaths; more over time.

CAUTION Avoid if you have high blood pressure or are pregnant.

mouth closed

hands, palms up, on your knees

sit cross-legged

01

Keeping your shoulders relaxed, inhale and exhale rapidly through the nose, which will produce a hissing sound. Breathe down into your belly.

03

Begin with 10 inhalations and exhalations per round. After the first round, allow your breathing to return to normal then complete 2 more rounds, pausing between them to breathe normally.

04

As you gain confidence, you can build up to more breaths per round, and also include a breath-retention process: after the last exhalation, take a deep nose breath and hold it for as long as is comfortable before exhaling.

05

When you feel ready, gently exhale through the nose and start breathing normally.

RESOURCES

Use these resources to find out more about breathwork
or find a practitioner, group or school in your area.

GLOBAL BREATHWORK ORGANIZATIONS

International Breathwork Foundation (IBF)
Global Inspiration Conference — **ibfnetwork.org**

Global Breathwork Professional Alliance (GBPA) — **breathworkalliance.com**

Breathing Circle Network — **breathingcircle.org**

SPECIFIC BREATH MODALITIES/TRAINING/ORGANIZATIONS

The following list offers a range of breathwork practices which you may feel inspired
to read about in more detail. It is not intended to be exhaustive and new practices are
evolving all the time. Each practice has specific attributes. Research different practices
until you find one that is suitable for your development. Always use discernment and
self-responsibility when choosing a therapist or group workshop leader.

Biodynamic Breath & Trauma Release System — **biodynamicbreath.com**

Bioenergetic Therapy – Alexander Lowen — **bioenergetic–therapy.com**

British Rebirth Society (BRS) — **rebirthingbreathwork.co.uk**

Buteyko Association — **buteykobreathing.org**

Clarity Breathwork — **claritybreathwork.com**

Coherent Breathing / Stephen Elliot — **coherence.com**

First–breath – Nathalia Westmacott–Brown — **first–breath.co.uk**

Holotropic Breathing / Dr. Stanislav Grof	**holotropic.com**
Holographic Breathing / Martin Jones	**holographic-breathing.com**
Hypnobirthing Breath	**thehypnobirthingassociation.com**
Integral Breath Therapy – Carol Lampman	**integrationconcepts.net**
Integrative Breathwork – Heinz & Lera Lange	**inbreath.org**
Liberation Breathing / Sondra Ray	**sondraray.com**
Middendorf Breathwork	**breathexperience.com**
Qigong / Dao Yin / Mantak Chia	**universal-tao.com**
Radiance Breathwork	**hendricks.com**
Reichian Breathwork	**reichianinstitute.org**
Rebirthing Breathwork / Leonard Orr	**rebirthingbreathwork.com**
Shamanic Breathwork	**shamanicbreathwork.org**
Somatic Breath Therapy	**powerofbreath.com**
Source Breathwork / Binny Dansby	**binnieadansby.com**
Spiritual Breathing / Dan Brûlée	**breathmastery.com**
Breathwork / Suta Guy Rawson	**tantricbreathwork.com**
Transformational Breathing / Dr. Judith Kravitz	**transformationalbreath.com**
Vivation Breathwork	**vivation.com**
Wim Hof® Method	**wimhofmethod.com**

INDEX

Index entries in **bold** indicate guided breathing exercises.

ABOUT THE AUTHOR

Nathalia Westmacott-Brown has been learning, practising, and teaching breathwork, since 2000. Her speciality is accessing pre-verbal experience, such as womb, birth and early infancy to work out how these early impressions impact our identity, breath and sense of self-esteem. She trained with a number of schools and International teachers and has blended these influences to create a unique approach of her own, which she now teaches to apprentice practitioners through her training organisation First-breath. She has years of involvement in global breathwork organisations, and has organised and delivered conferences in both the UK and India. Nathalia has travelled extensively with the Global Inspiration Conference to experience first-hand the most inspiring teachers and methods around the world. In 2008 she founded the worldwide breathing initiative "Breathing Circle" which promotes a monthly breathing event in 24 different countries. She lives with her home-schooled daughter Iris and a menagerie of rescued animals in an apple orchard in Worcestershire, England.

AUTHOR'S ACKNOWLEDGMENTS

It is a privilege to write a book on Breathwork, a practice which has drastically transformed my life. I am in awe of the process and grateful to the pioneers, teachers and initiates who have gone before. These ancestors are the foundation of modern-day breathwork. Likewise, I am deeply appreciative to my own spiritual teachers, specifically my mentor, Christina Artemis, who introduced me to this treasured path, many moons ago. Thank you also to my dear friend Clare Gabriel, who inspired me to take a deep breath and jump. I feel gratitude to my breathwork colleagues, who offered practices from their own traditions for inclusion in this book. For the love, encouragement and quiet spaces to write, I thank my friends and family, especially Sam, Christina, Julia, Elfi and Andy who provided love and sandwiches. Most of all, to my husband Pete & my daughter Iris, it was your love, patience and wisdom that helped me to 'birth' this little book into being. Finally, love and respect to the DK team Lesley, Rona and Dawn, who know a raw diamond when they see one. Thank you for the opportunity to shine.

PUBLISHER'S ACKNOWLEDGMENTS

DK would like to thank the following people for their assistance in the publication of this book: Clare Gabriel for helping with the early conception of the book, Keith Hagan for illustration assistance, John Friend for proofreading, and Marie Lorimer for compiling the index.